Love
Healing
Forgiveness
Peace
Joy

REGINA CHOUZA

A Personal Guide to Self-Healing, Cancer and Love

REGINA CHOUZA

DISCLAIMER

This book gives non-specific, general advice and should not be relied on as a substitute for proper medical care and consultation. Reiki, Energy Healing and meditation are complementary therapies. They are not intended to replace conventional medical care. If you have an acute or chronic disease you should consult a qualified health care professional.

While all suggested Self-Healing techniques are offered in good faith, the author and publisher accept no liability for damage of any nature resulting directly or indirectly from the application or use of information in this book, or from the failure to seek medical advice from a doctor.

Website: www.diaryofapsychichealer.com

ISBN: 978-1484930601

This book is dedicated
to "Alejandro papá"

Contents

Acknowledgments

Preface   Pg 1

Introduction   Pg 7

Part I   Why Do People Get Sick?   Pg 11

    Chapter 1:   Risk Factors for Disease   Pg 12

    Chapter 2:   What Can We Learn by Being Sick?   Pg 29

Part II   Introduction to Energy Healing   Pg 37

    Chapter 3:   The Energy Body   Pg 41

    Chapter 4:   Self-Healing Techniques   Pg 49

    Chapter 5:   What Do Energy Healers Do?   Pg 59

    Chapter 6:   Energy Healing for The Family   Pg 64

    Epilogue :   Examining Your Beliefs   Pg 72

Appendix 1 :   Guided Meditations   Pg 75

Appendix 2 :   Glossary   Pg 87

Appendix 3 :   Energy Management for Beginners   Pg 89

Appendix 4 :   Recommended Reading   Pg 93

REGINA CHOUZA

Acknowledgements

Self-publishing this book turned out to be a much bigger piece of work than I ever anticipated, though thankfully we never go it alone. My deepest gratitude goes to the editorial angels who were incredibly generous with their time and energy: Gail Le Breton, who reviewed the early drafts and helped me shape this book; Tara Flanagan, whose attention to detail, generosity and editing skills have saved me from publishing a decidedly home-cooked book; Kim Liebenberg and Leslie Sommers for having one last look before it went to print; and Wocjiech "Nathaniel" Ucarzewics for converting this to an e-book. And of course, Adrian Lui and the rest of the team at Amazon for making self-publishing user friendly.

Finding the time and energy to write a book can be one of the biggest obstacles. I am incredibly grateful to Vivan Pinto, Sandra Chatelain, Esther O'Reilly and Kate Ashton for facilitating my transition out of the corporate world and making this book project possible. Sharing the first drafts was nerve wracking though I was lucky to receive honest, constructive feedback from Sasha Begum, Alejandra Ponce, Maria Veiga, Anne Evans, Vanessa Stoecklein, Rachel Cooper, and of course, my healing tutor Sharon Holmes. Without their support it would have been much harder to find the courage to finish the job. I would also like to thank Shaza Al-Sabban for patiently answering questions on genetics as well as Justin Bonnet and Matina Vidalis for being brilliant sounding boards.

As a child I dreamt of writing a book and Energy Healing has finally given me something worthwhile to write about. I was very lucky to meet a talented group of healing tutors when I moved to London four years ago: Natasha Wojnow whose "Could I be a Healer?" course first piqued my interest; Sue Allen, Sharon Holmes and Julia Shepherd at the School of Intuition and Healing; and Amanda Roberts and Michelle Hawcroft at the College of Psychic Studies. And last but not least, Michael Kaufmann whose fluid approach has made Reiki thoroughly enjoyable. My blog readers and Facebook fans have also been a great source of inspiration. I feel blessed to swap stories with a this lovely group who remind me that there is still so much to be learned and explored. Thank you for your constant enthusiasm!

The cover design process was one of the most enjoyable parts of this project, thanks to the talented Cati Sarquis who created loads of beautiful designs, and to my real-life and Facebook friends who weighed in on the options. Especially my former colleagues at J&J: Sudarshana Sinha, Diana Cuturela, Sarah Brown, Sissel Gynnild, Rebecca Lutwyche, James Fulton, Francesco Salvo di Pietraganzilli, Sandra Chatelain, Alexandra Papas, Louise Bradley and Charlotte Ridley. A special thank you goes to the Diary of a Psychic Healer Facebook Page for voting on cover designs and for prompting me to choose starry Chakras. I cannot begin to tell you how encouraging it has been to share my experiences with such an enthusiastic group over the past three years. Thousands of angels will get their wings!

My heartfelt gratitude goes to my family who has been an invaluable source of support since the word cancer first came onto the scene: Tatiz, Ma, Eloy, Anilu, Bea, Gustavo, Ricardo, Susana, Paulina, Jose Luis, Mari, Federico, Pati, Agustin, Ramon, Nora, Zarco, Yamel, Eva, Julian, Lupita, *las tias* Pati y Tere, *mis primos y muchos mas.* Also to our extended family and lifelong friends including: Fernando y Marcela, Gaston y Mercedes, Enrique, and the Martin del Campo, Perez Simon, Guichard and Mauser clans. To my Boston friends who were a rock in the not-so-good-old days: especially Sasha Begum, Alejandra Ponce, Aline Pitanga, and Cassandra Longoria; and finally to Guiso, Daniela, Kato and Fernando for bringing a breath of fresh air to our modern family.

Lastly, I would not be writing this book without a lifetime of unconditional love, support and encouragement from my parents, Jennie and Alejandro, and my siblings Alejandro, Ximena and Mafer. This is as much their story as it is mine.

Preface

Although I did not know it at the time, the winter of 1996 would change my life forever. My family lived in La Jolla, California. I was 16 and had just returned home after a year in boarding school. La Jolla was a beautiful place full of sunshine, weekends at the beach and tennis clubs. My brother was back from a year in military school and our younger sisters were both in elementary school. On the surface everything looked the same but life was slowly starting to change. Our dad traveled for work regularly and we were used to seeing him on weekends. His work was winding down and though he had more time to spend with us, he never seemed to have the energy for it. In the space of a year he had gone from being playful and good-natured to volatile, stubborn and always tired. He complained of nausea and headaches, but migraines run in the family so we did not think much of it. I remember being pissed off one weekend when he would not get up off the couch. We were running late for a special occasion. I thought something along the lines of "It's not like you have cancer," and stomped off.

At times it was as if I had come home to a stranger. Dad, at age 45, was acting erratically, camping out in pajamas and watching TV all day. I thought it was delayed grief over my grandfather's death a few years earlier. The two of them never got along. *Abuelo*, Spanish for grandfather, had a difficult upbringing and he carried the scars with him through life. Growing up, Dad felt torn between forced loyalty to Abuelo and his love for the maternal grandfather who always reached out to him. That conflict was one

1

of the reasons why my parents moved to California shortly after I was born. The last years of Abuelo's life were full of drama, emotional tension and what soon became a feud between father and son. In retrospect, Dad would have benefited from counseling to deal with the emotional turmoil and to see Abuelo in a more forgiving light. Instead, Dad swept it under the rug. With this history bubbling under the surface, it was not surprising to see it play out as apathy, depression and frequent migraines.

Dad was increasingly hard to live with and eventually he decided to live part-time at my grandmother's summerhouse nearby. He came and went between the two homes, much like he had commuted to Mexico City for the better part of five years. That December we spent Christmas Eve together at home and had planned a skiing holiday in Colorado. But Dad came down with the flu and we left without him. He promised to fly out when he felt better, but the days went by and he had no plans to join us. My mom was worried because he did not sound like himself. We felt disconnected and helpless, staying in a small ski lodge hundreds of miles away. My mom rang her best friend, Cristina, who we knew as *La Teacher* because she gave private cooking lessons in the area. She and her husband lived off the San Diego coast on beautiful Coronado Island.

Mom was reluctant to ask the favor as it meant a 40-minute drive from Coronado to La Jolla. Better safe than sorry. Cristina packed a sandwich and sent her husband, Guillermo, to check on Dad. He rang the doorbell and got no response. Guillermo cracked open a side window, removed the mosquito net and climbed through. Dad was on the second floor watching television. He heard the doorbell but did not think to answer it. Guillermo made small talk while my dad ate the sandwich. He seemed OK but the days went by and Dad still felt unwell. This time my dad's older brother went to check on him. He decided to take him to the hospital. How my uncle managed to get him down the stairs we will never know! At six feet five and 220 pounds, my dad was a big guy. Luckily, so was my uncle. The thought of them stumbling to the car made us chuckle a few days later.

My uncle rang from the hospital to let us know what was happening. Something about a CAT scan. The word was familiar because I had heard it on the television show, *ER*. He promised to call when there was news. It was just after midnight when the phone rang again. All I remember was my mom crying when she heard the news. Dad had a malignant brain tumor. It was big – roughly the size of an orange. Were it not for the trip to the hospital, Dad might not have made it through the weekend. Looking back on it, we were extremely lucky that he stayed behind that December. One of the country's top neurosurgeons worked at the local hospital. Dad was prepped for surgery that week. I do not know what would have happened if they had discovered the tumor in a ski resort, just days after Christmas.

We flew back to San Diego the next morning. I do not remember much of what happened that week; only that the pumpernickel bread in the hospital cafeteria was tasty. We spent five days at Scripps Memorial Hospital before and after the surgery. My family is originally from Mexico and the waiting room looked like a scene from a movie because we had so many friends camping out in the hallways. The hospital staff had to tell us to keep our visitor numbers down, but it was incredibly helpful to have so many loved ones supporting us. The surgery went well, thanks to the brilliant surgical team who got 98 percent of the tumor in just four hours. The recovery also seemed easier than any of us expected. Two weeks later, Dad was cheering at my sister's soccer game. I kept telling him to sit down, and needless to say, his "header" jokes were not funny! We were relieved to put the surgery behind us. But there was still a silent cloud over our heads.

Dad had several radiotherapy treatments over the next few months. Eventually his doctors suggested a special laser surgery to get the last of it. I did not know it at the time, but there was a good chance the tumor would return. At that point the doctors put his life expectancy at nine months. We packed our bags and moved to Mexico City, where our extended family lived. Lucky for us, life expectancy estimates are only based on statistics.

A year went by and he was still perfectly healthy. I went off to college in Boston and my brother returned to the US for college a year later. We had a quiet New Years in San Diego that year with La Teacher and Guillermo, two years after the scare in the hospital. By then Dad was taking an interest in life, planning holidays to Europe and coming up with new business ideas. He was happy, playful and enthusiastic, going on and on about a franchise business that he wanted to set up. One day I asked him why he had not put his business plan into practice. He said he was waiting for the five-year mark. Until then there was still a risk that the cancer might come back. He did not want to leave us saddled with a fledgling business. I think that might have been the only time he mentioned it. All in all, we had four good years without any mention of the word *cancer*.

The health scare pushed him to broaden his horizons. For nearly a decade we had been taking the same holidays: summers in Mexico City and winters in Colorado. We went skiing one more time and then decided not to go back. It had gotten old. We spent the next holidays in Paris, my Dad's favorite city, before traveling to Italy and Spain with my grandmother, aunts, uncles and cousins. It was a trip down memory lane for my dad and my uncles, who had lived in Spain as teenagers. We had a lot of laughs, especially when a fancy restaurant sent a roasted pheasant, head intact, to the table on New Year's Eve. My sisters, aged 10 and 12, screamed bloody murder as soon as they caught the look of agony on the bird's face. Dad covered its head with a napkin, which did not help, and eventually the bird went back to the kitchen. Even today, the memory still makes me laugh.

The next summer, however, Dad went in for his six-month checkup and a tumor appeared on the scans. It was small and we were optimistic about catching it early. He had surgery again, and this time the doctors got it all. The surgeon suggested a follow-up six weeks later, but we were not worried about it. I flew back to school in Boston, my sister left for boarding school, and my brother went to Italy on his semester abroad. Only my mom and my youngest sister stayed behind for the recovery. The surgery had gone well and we expected to put it behind us. It was my senior year of college and life was pretty normal. The main exception was Sept. 11 and the chaos that ensued. Dad woke me up calling to see if I was okay. How ironic! He had just been through brain surgery two weeks earlier. I should have been worried about him, not the other way around!

My parents went back to the hospital for a scan the first week of October. They expected to go back together for the results three days later. But the surgeon rang my mother the next morning and told her to come around by herself. It was dreadful news. Though the surgery had removed the tumor completely, there was a new one in a different part of his brain. It was too soon after the surgery to operate again and even if it were possible, we could expect more to come. There was nothing he could do about it. Dad's case was terminal. My mom called that evening to soften the blow before giving us the full news a few days later. It was a real shock. After four years and nine months we had reached the end of the line. We were in a state of disbelief and my dad, for one, never acknowledged the prognosis. This made the next few months even harder, though we had to respect his wishes. I can only imagine how he must have felt when he heard the news.

My brother and I flew home immediately. We did not know how long he had. Maybe three months, maybe a year. Dad's health deteriorated rapidly. My sister came home Dec. 15 and Dad slipped into a coma the next day. Mom had a grief counselor come to see us that week. That was a conversation I never expected to have. The counselor told us what to expect in the last few weeks. For example, we might feel relief when it was finally over. She told us it was normal to wish the end would come sooner. That was hard to hear, but she was right. In those last days we also worried about practical considerations. For example, pain medication was in short supply in pharmacies. We were constantly on the phone to local drugstores and wound up buying the medication straight from a wholesaler.

Our expectations for Christmas were low that year but we managed to have a pleasant time. My aunts, uncles and cousins came over for dinner. It was a welcome break from the steady stream of nurses and others who added to the emotional overload in the house. Dad passed away a few days later – five years to the day of his initial diagnosis in the ER. The irony was not lost on us; we saw it as an extension on his life. My feelings were a mix of relief, sadness and disbelief at his passing, as well as gratitude for five years that were, for the most part, happy.

We were also relieved that it was quick and relatively painless. Cancer can be a harsh disease and we wanted him at peace more than anything else. When my brother and I walked past a pharmacy the following week we both remarked that our first thought was whether they had painkillers in stock. I could not help smiling. It finally dawned on me that we did not have to worry anymore and a huge weight came off my shoulders.

Looking back on it, I have learned a lot from the experience.

I have deep respect for the medical profession and I am grateful to the wonderful doctors, nurses and technicians who treated my dad. Their dedication, skill and expertise gave him the best chance of survival. That said, for nearly four years, he was their miracle case. At one point, the radiotherapy team greeted him with tears in their eyes. They never expected him to make it for so long. The fact that he outlived their expectations by four years, and then passed on the same calendar day of his initial diagnosis tells me someone upstairs is in charge.

One of the theories of Energy Healing states that illness often follows a strong emotional upset in a person's life. It might be the loss of a job, a divorce or in my dad's case, a massive falling out in the family. I have always had the intuitive knowledge that my dad's cancer was connected to the fight with Abuelo. I just did not know how. If I had to hazard a guess, I would say that the brain tumor represented his inability to see past the fight with Abuelo. Holding a grudge will eat away at a person from the inside, much like a cancer. How does this relate to his tumor? Is it possible that forgiving my grandfather would have helped?

The illness put an enormous strain on the family but in retrospect, we gained a lot from it. Dad's job required lots of travel and we were starting to drift apart. After the surgery he had to cut back on his work hours and this gave us time with him. The five years were a blessing, especially for my sisters who were eight and ten when he first got sick. They got to spend quality time with him before he passed away. Those years were a gift for everyone but especially for my sisters.

Introduction

When I started writing this book my intent was to create an Energy Healing guide for cancer patients. The idea was to share my family's experience – how it changed our lives and the perspective I have gained since then through my own healing journey. I also wanted to give others a chance to apply the techniques learned during a two-year healing course at the School of Intuition and Healing in London. Since then, this project has evolved into much more, no doubt thanks to my background in philosophy which means I enjoy asking questions. The first half of the book explores the question "Why do people get sick?" from biological and spiritual points of view. I cover a variety of factors ranging from diet, genetics and lifestyle to emotional and mental patterns that may hold back the healing process. I also believe that every difficult experience gives us valuable insights and lessons. Cancer is no exception. Some may feel regret over the direction they have taken with their lives and how much quality time they have spent with family and friends. The healing process involves accepting these feelings when they arise, learning from them and moving on.

The second half of the book explores Energy Healing as a complementary therapy to medical intervention. Energy Healing is a broad term that can be used to describe a variety of self-healing techniques including guided meditations, breathing exercises, journaling and hands-on healing such as Reiki. My theory is that Energy Healing addresses the mental, emotional and spiritual aspects of disease while medical intervention treats the physical body. These two disciplines can work together. This book will give the a reader a basic understanding of the energy body, including the Aura and the Chakras, and how we can use a variety of self-healing techniques to release stress, tension and even old hurts and beliefs that may be undermining the healing process. Because these techniques also help manage mental and emotional stress, which can easily leave a person feeling drained, Energy Healing can be useful for the whole family.

My approach to Energy Healing hinges on the belief that our thoughts, emotions and reactions have an emotional charge. A positive experience can leave you feeling happy and energized. A negative experience does the opposite. For example, a severe disappointment can leave a person feeling angry, bewildered or hurt. Self-healing involves releasing these emotions from our consciousness and moving on. Some people find it easy to forgive. Others have trouble letting go, especially when there is a genuine grievance to overcome. Healing techniques facilitate the process, but ultimately it is the individual who lets go. Energy Healing can also help manage feelings of anxiety, hopelessness, anger and resentment. The last two can be especially toxic. I believe that with time, buried resentment and anger will eat away at a person from the inside, much like a tumor, and that for healing to occur on all four levels – mental, emotional, spiritual and physical – we need to connect with the energy of unconditional love and forgiveness. Hence the title of this book: *Self-Healing, Cancer & Love.*

Earlier I stated that Energy Healing is complementary to medical care. This is a legal requirement in some countries and I agree wholeheartedly for the following reasons:

1. Even if we could prove that anger and resentment are at the root of most cancer cases, it may be easier to have surgery than it is to genuinely forgive.

2. I have not seen robust evidence to show that healing alone, or any complementary therapy by itself will prolong a cancer patient's life. Individual case studies do not have the statistical significance to predict an outcome. Rather, that statistical confidence can only be found in

randomized control trials, where large patient groups are administered one of several treatment options under medical supervision.

3. Though we would certainly like to, the role of the energy healer is not to save the client's life. We are there to facilitate their self-healing process and their soul path. Energy Healing will not save a client from a learning experience that they are meant to have. In some cases, the illness may be necessary to trigger a change of consciousness before the patient moves on to the next stage in their life. For others, it may be their time to go and Energy Healing can help them find comfort and peace.

REGINA CHOUZA

Part I
Why Do People Get Sick?

Chapter 1

Risk Factors for Disease

When I started writing this book, I made a list of reasons why people might get sick. There were several risk factors on the list: diet, lack of exercise, stress, genetics and obesity. I also had a shorter list of things that we stand to gain when we are ill, though they cannot be described as risk factors. They include attention, time off work and feeling cared for. This got me thinking: Can we divide the list into risk factors and potential benefits? A risk factor is a pre-existing condition that makes it more likely for a person to fall ill. A benefit could be a positive side effect, usually mental, emotional or spiritual. I do not think people get sick on purpose but there is something to be learned from every difficult experience. For example, hard times can teach us to be compassionate. They also can be a reminder of what is most important in life, prompting us to rethink our priorities and live a life that is more aligned to our authentic spirits.

Risk factors can be used to identify groups of people who might be at risk, but they cannot predict if a disease will manifest. Each type of cancer also has its own set of risk factors to consider. For example, sun exposure is relevant to skin cancer, but not to lung and mouth cancer, which are linked to smoking. In this book I have focused on risk factors which are relevant on a wider scale. However, there are still lots of grey areas that need to be accounted for, as this quote from Cancer.org shows:

"Most women who have one or more breast cancer risk factors never develop the disease, while many women with breast cancer have no apparent risk factors (other than being a woman and growing older). Even when a woman with risk factors develops breast cancer, it is hard to know just how much these factors might have contributed."[1]

I believe there are also emotional and energetic risk factors, which could help us explain the grey areas. In this book I will discuss several aspects that may influence cancer. Though these may apply to any illness, I believe them to be particularly relevant for cancer patients.

One of my dad's friends is a research oncologist. A few years after Dad passed away, he came to visit us with his wife and kids. It was nice to see them and we spent a lot of time talking about the good old days. Eventually the topic turned to his job and the research he was doing. His focus is primarily on chemotherapy treatments that are less stressful for patients. I thought it was remarkable that he was dedicating his life to making cancer treatments less of a burden for patients. The conversation eventually turned to my dad's case and how young he was when he was diagnosed with cancer. We went on to talk about cancer incidence in general and what might be accountable for the statistics.

His answer was simple: nutrition.

Diet and Exercise

My dad's friend had been analyzing the incidence of cancer in different countries. He remarked on the cultural differences between them and how their lifestyle might lead to certain types of cancer. For example, the Western world consumes large amounts of processed and microwavable food. Obesity, a big risk factor for cancer, is closely linked to diet and exercise. Cancer incidence was on the rise for decades, until awareness made prevention possible for certain types of cancer. Inversely, Japan had

---

[1] American Cancer Society: Breast Cancer: Accessed March 2013.
http://www.cancer.org/cancer/breastcancer/detailedguide/breast-cancer-risk-factors

historically low rates of cancer, the main exception being the incidence of stomach cancer. He attributed the differences to the Japanese diet, which is typically healthier, though it is unusually high in pickled foods. Research has also linked the elevated salt content in the Japanese diet (soy sauce) to acute gastritis, a potential risk factor for stomach and gastric cancers[2]. In an otherwise healthy diet, these exceptions make a difference. Though I am not an expert on nutrition or dietary advice, common sense tells me that eating fresh and organic foods like chicken, fish, fruits and vegetables is conducive to good health. This would also help keep obesity rates in check.

Alcohol Consumption

A few years ago I went to see a movie by the name of *La Môme*, based on Edith Piaf's life. Ms. Piaf was a celebrated French singer also known for her rough lifestyle. The movie portrayed her partying hard: smoking, drinking and running her body into the ground. By the time the character turned 45, the actress hunched over like an old woman. I was curious about her health and looked for information online. It turns out she was diagnosed with lung cancer in her forties. My first reaction was to criticize the filmmakers for making it seem like her health was due to excessive smoking and drinking. Why didn't they say she had cancer? I mentioned this to a friend, who remarked that her lifestyle might have caused the cancer. The thought had not occurred to me. Since then I have had the chance to learn more about the effects of cigarettes and alcohol.

When the human body digests the alcohol in beer, wine and other liquors, it transforms the ethanol content into a carcinogenic enzyme known as acetaldehyde. Acetaldehyde (AA) is naturally present in the body and in many foods. The body can metabolize a certain amount of AA without it posing a health risk. The problem comes when the body has more AA than it can process and it finds its way into the bloodstream. This in turn exposes tissues throughout the body to AA. It poses a serious health risk for societies where drinking over the limit is common.

---

[2] National Institute of Health: Gut. 2006 November; 55(11): 1545–1552.
http://www.ncbi.nlm.nih.gov/pmc/articles/PMC1860129/

Cigarette Smoking

Inhaling smoke on a daily basis is bad enough for the lungs, but smoking also adds to the levels of acetaldehyde in the body. This means that smoking could lead to cancer anywhere in the body. Secondhand smoke has the same effect. You will find infinite information on the dangers of smoking, but there is also plenty of support out there for those who want to quit. In addition, clearing and healing the Sacral Chakra can help with addictions. Please keep this in mind during healing meditations. If quitting is too much to aim for, cutting back should also reduce the amount of acetaldehyde in the body. Every little bit helps!

Stress and Tension

Stress and tension are big drivers for dis-ease in the human body. I spell disease with a hyphen because illness pushes the body out of balance so that we are no longer comfortable in our own skin. Stress is quick to do this. Some people may start to experience loss of hair, sweating, weight loss, compulsive over eating, ulcers and tension headaches or backaches. It is also known to lower our natural defenses, which can make the body more vulnerable. Is it possible that prolonged exposure to stress may cause cancer? When I first published this book in the year 2013 I didn't have a scientific answer to this question, but my intuition loudly said YES.

Since then, the *University of Montreal* has conducted research into perceived work related stress over the span of decades and the link it has with various types of cancer. While the study focused on the risk associated with specific high intensity jobs, prolonged exposure (15+ years) to work-related stress was linked to increased risk of lung, colon, rectal and stomach cancer as well as non-Hodgkin lymphoma in men[3]. The study assessed a number of factors including job security, financial troubles, tough commutes and risks to personal safety. While further research is needed to understand the influence across larger population groups, these findings indicate a need for effective stress relief tools as well as psychological

---

[3] Lifetime report of perceived stress at work & cancer among men: A case-control study in Montreal, Canada. Audrey Blanc-Lapierre, Marie Claude Rousseau, Deborah Weiss, et al.

support from employers. Who knows, we may have good reason to ask for standard mental health days, or paid leave for workers in certain industries!

When we come onto the subject of genetics I will also discuss how a stressful lifestyle can compound genetic risk factors. Relaxation techniques are all the more valuable if we think about healing from this perspective.

Depression and Grief

One of my professors in business school used to joke that alcohol is stronger when a person has just been through a breakup. The class laughed off his comment but I think he had a point. When a person's emotional health and state of mind suffer, their defenses go down and it makes it easier for things like bacteria and viruses to infiltrate the body. It also has an effect on our energetic boundaries, which serve to protect our space and also to contain our personal energy. If a person is depressed, these boundaries weaken and their personal energy escapes. Low energy levels lead to fatigue, a weak immune system, and even weaker boundaries. With time this depletes a person's energy.

Depression is said to precede the onset of illnesses like cancer. Whether it causes cancer is a different matter – one I do not know the answer to. But just think of the implications: A person with low energy levels is suddenly faced with aggressive treatments that further deplete their personal energy. Looking after the entire body can be extremely helpful. This is why I believe energy healing complements medical treatments, whether it is a hands-on-healing session or a meditation that we opt for.

Grief has a similar effect on the body, bringing emotions such as anger, confusion, denial, acute stress and shock into the mix. Intuitive Healers are taught to ask about a person's life in the years leading up to a cancer diagnosis. Based on anecdotal evidence, Healers operate under the assumption that grief is a risk factor for cancer. For example, were there upheavals in their personal, professional or family lives? How did they cope with the loss of their home or the death of a loved one - and are those emotions still raw? In these cases, one would complement conventional medical care with emotional healing to release the energy of grief, anger or pain from the body, using the tools in Chapters 4 through 6.

Anecdotal evidence is not likely to sway the scientific community on the subject of emotional risk factors, as individual case studies do not have the statistical significance to predict an outcome. Rather, that confidence can be found in randomized control trials (RCT's) where large patients groups are observed methodically and objectively. This is why a recent study at *Peking Union Medical College* is so promising. A systematic review of multiple RCT's has found a potential link between "striking life events" and primary breast cancer in women. These events were defined to include the death of a family member, divorce, financial troubles, retirement, unemployment and relocation. While the researchers do indicate the need for more research into the connection between acute stress, grief and cancer, they also conclude that "women with striking life events were at 1.5-fold higher risk of developing breast cancer than women without…[4]"

Given these findings, it is crucial to make self-healing a part of our daily lives. Ideally the self-healing journey would begin when the striking life event takes place – in which case we could approach emotional healing from a cancer prevention point of view. If the person has already been diagnosed with cancer then more pressing considerations take precedence. Introducing the subject of emotional risk factors at that point may add confusion to an already overwhelming situation. Once the medical emergency has been addressed, the patient will once again have the frame of mind for introspection and emotional healing. In the short term, the priority should be placed on medical intervention and stress relief techniques to help them through the physical crisis. As an energy healer or Reiki practitioner, it is possible to send healing to the memory and to the pain it caused, without asking the patient to relive the situation yet again.

Note: While this systematic review indicates a link between 'striking life events' and breast cancer, we cannot assume that emotional healing will be enough to treat the disease. Instead, we can use this information to direct our energy healing sessions while taking a compassionate approach with the patient - who is now going through another life

---

[4] Yan Lin. Striking life events associated with primary breast cancer susceptibility in women: a meta-analysis study." Journal of Experimental & Clinical Cancer Research 2013.

event. The subject of emotional risk factors is often difficult to raise because it can be misunderstood as 'blaming the patient' for being angry or hurt and not letting go, when in reality, they need love, compassion and understanding. How many of us would react to the above mentioned 'striking life events' with complete peace and harmony? Not many...

Heredity and The Cancer Gene

Most of us are familiar with genetics. Our family's medical history can tell us whether we are at risk of heart attacks, diabetes, high blood pressure and also less threatening conditions like hair loss. Is it possible for cancer to run in the family as well? The question first crossed my mind in the 1990's when three relatives on my dad's side of the family were diagnosed with cancer. Was it bad luck, genetics or something else? The truth is cancer genes do exist, but as I have learned, we need to see two people on the same side of the family with the same type of cancer for it to be genetic. Even then it may be possible to reduce the likelihood of a disease gene expressing itself yet again. Hopefully the following insights will reduce the sense of inevitability around genetics. It is also important to remember that each case is unique. The fact that a relative was not able to heal from cancer has no bearing on their niece, their child or their brother's chances.

In this book I have focused on risk factors that can be minimized by modifying lifestyle and habits. This holds true for genetics. Research indicates that obesity genes are less likely to express themselves as disease if we pay attention to nutrition and exercise. A single workout has an immediate effect, reducing obesity mRNA levels by 30%. The mRNA molecule plays a vital role in gene expression, copying DNA and making it available to the cells. A daily exercise regime reduced these levels by nearly half in four weeks, though they also revert to neutral after a day of rest[5].

This knowledge is especially relevant now that DNA testing is becoming more and more accessible to the general public. In all likelihood, many of us are predisposed to at least one illness. The question is, how do you live with that knowledge? If a woman carries breast cancer gene mutations Brca1 or Brca2, the risk is high and her doctor may suggest preventative surgery, regardless of lifestyle habits. Regular screening will

---

[5] The Effect of Exercise on ob Gene Expression. Dongai Zeng. 1996.

also be an option for these and other types of cancer. Only your doctor can advise on your genetic makeup and the risk it carries, though it will be empowering to know that a healthy lifestyle may very well offset that risk.

Though we cannot change our DNA sequence, research indicates that living a healthy lifestyle can put genes for certain illnesses into "sleep mode," making it less likely for them to manifest in your lifetime, *and potentially in the next generation's.* These findings are part of a new branch of science known as epigenetics. Most of us are familiar with the human genome, the DNA spiral that sits at the core of every last cell in your body. It holds an infinite number of possible physical traits: mom's blue eyes, dad's full head of hair, grandpa's receding hairline, grandma's gene for obesity – the list goes on and on. How do our cells know which genes to express? That is where the epigenome comes into a play: a thin layer of chemical proteins that cover the DNA spiral.

The epigenome is full of chemical imprints, data points if you will, that tell the DNA in each cell what to become. For example, it might indicate that a cell will be part of a yellow speck in a blue iris. The human body is constantly replenishing cells. New cells inherit the old cells' epigenetic markers, ensuring consistency and continuity in the body. This lesson in genetics is relevant because lifestyle factors such as stress, diet, alcohol and smoking leave a mark on the epigenome. Logically, it would follow that prolonged stress levels will have a cumulative effect on the epigenome. How that translates to cell replication has yet to be seen, though intuitively you would think that *reducing* these stressors should have a positive effect[6].

Research indicates that epigenetic markers can be passed down from parent to child; if dad's obesity gene was silenced, his children may inherit the epigenetic markers that silenced that gene. Let's hope the mother also leads a healthy lifestyle as kids get half of their markers from each parent.

Epigenetics is still in its infancy and it may be too soon to speculate on the interaction between specific cancer genes, the epigenome and environmental factors such as stress, smoking or alcohol. The

---

[6] Science Museum; Who am I? Accessed in November 2012.
http://www.sciencemuseum.org.uk/WhoAmI/FindOutMore/Yourgenes.aspx

pharmaceutical industry is said to be researching the topic in the hopes of developing drugs that could silence disease genes through the epigenome. Drugs aside, what can we do in the meantime to help? My intuition suggests that we start by modifying known lifestyle factors: Follow a healthy diet, exercise and cut back on alcohol and cigarette smoking. The other big culprit is stress. Relaxation techniques may have a direct impact on your physical health as well as boosting your state of mind. Find a relaxation technique you enjoy; there are plenty to choose from including meditation, conscious breathing, yoga and of course, Reiki and Energy Healing.

Let's not forget that we can also act on the stress triggers. Stress is linked to fear, such as missing a deadline or not being able to pay the rent. Improving your organizational skills, learning to ask for help and clearing your mind will help reduce stress levels on a daily basis.

Memetics: Learned Behaviors in The Family Tree

Memetics first caught my attention in the fall of 2001. At the time I was a senior at Tufts University, just about ready to wrap up my undergraduate degree in Philosophy. One of my professors was writing a book on evolutionary biology. We covered several topics that year but one stayed with me: meme replication. If genes are part of our biological makeup, memes are part of our behavioral DNA. They are the behavioral patterns that we adopt through imitation. Memes often spread across entire cultures and nationalities, accounting for some of the cultural stereotypes we have today. What makes Americans individualistic, Mexicans welcoming and relaxed and the French a little bit stubborn? These and other cultural traits are transmitted through meme replication. With time they might even become part of our cultural identity – how we distinguish ourselves.

The memes that survive often have a strong psychological or emotional charge. A family's sense of identity is often characterized by these traits. For example, children might grow up hearing that they are "their mother's child" because they have the same stubborn streak. They grow up thinking it is part of their nature and they are unapologetic about it. It reinforces the family bond. This is harmless when memes are positive; for example, adopting a healthy work ethic. But other memes can hold a person back. For example, the tendency to see yourself as a victim may prevent you from taking responsibility for your life. Some people learn to shift blame onto others. They wind up in a vicious circle where things go bad and they point fingers rather than finding a solution. The tendency toward violence is also a meme. A person may have learned to stifle his emotions and find an outlet in violent rages. All of these memes have consequences. Positive ones enrich relationships and experiences by providing a healthy attitude. Unhealthy memes sabotage your relationships, your career and even your health.

The learned behaviors relevant to healing influence our interactions with others. Every interaction has an energetic charge that increases, decreases or maintains your personal energy levels. Overly generous souls may find themselves in a constant giving mode. Though they do this gladly, perhaps even compulsively, giving too much of themselves can deplete their energy levels.

It may start as a recurring tiredness. Unchecked it becomes fatigue, and if they feel compelled to keep on giving, their defenses may become so depleted that they fall ill. In *Extraordinary Psychic,* Deborah Lynn Katz tells us that many compulsive healers risk depleting their Heart Chakras, putting themselves at risk of breast cancer. The Heart Chakra and the breasts are both related to the nurturing and mothering aspect. Over-nurturing clients, children or friends can deplete the Healer's (or the mother's) energy. That imbalance manifests as a disease, and in this case breast cancer has been signaled out as the likely candidate.

The Body Holds on to Unresolved Emotional Issues

It is more or less accepted that the human body feels the tension of our fast-paced lives. Everyone reacts to stress, tension and pressures in their own way. Some people let go of steam by going for a run or to the gym. Others meditate. Still others tense their shoulders, back and jaw without noticing. They internalize that nervous tension. These muscles can even remain in a state of constant tension. Prolonged stress can lead to chronic back pain, hair loss and even ulcers. The degree to which we are able to handle stress determines our quality of life and our relationships. Thinking ahead, improving our organizational skills and getting a good night's sleep can reduce situational stress. Exercise, meditation and other relaxation techniques can also help release stress and tension from the human body.

It is important to note that stress is an underlying feeling or emotion. It is not an event, a deadline, or a bill. Stress is the state of nervous tension that arises when we are faced with fear, often in response to fear of failure. For example, failing to pass an exam, failing to meet a deadline, etc. Fear leads to stress and if this is not released from the body it may cause medical conditions such as chronic back pain and even ulcers. According to Energy Healing, this happens when fear has become trapped in the muscles or the digestive system. In Chapter 4, I will discuss self-healing techniques that can be used to release emotions like fear from the body. For now, let's focus on how this happens and why it matters.

When people have trouble letting go of emotions like anger, resentment or jealousy, these emotions are also stored in their organs. As an intuitive healer, I sometimes notice this in a client's body. It might come across as a feeling of sadness lingering over a particular organ. In one instance I was prompted to send healing to a client's pancreas. I sensed resentment in his pancreas and got the intuitive feeling that it was directed at a parent. There were also traces of betrayal, anger and grief. I did not know what had happened between them. After the session, I asked the client about his relationship with his parents and his response pointed to the father. Since then we have used the healing sessions to release these emotions from his energy field. The wound is recent and it has not had an effect on his physical body. It may never come to that.

It is important to remember that everyone goes through loss, disappointment or grief at some point in life. This is not about pointing fingers at the person who caused the pain. What matters is how we react and whether we are able to heal and move on. Some people are comfortable talking about their feelings. They let go of the past by speaking to a counselor, by crying on a friend's shoulder or by confronting the person who hurt them. Others find creative outlets for their grief: singing, dancing, writing, painting. Left alone, anger often turns to resentment, an emotion that will eat away at a person from the inside. As mentioned earlier, I believe buried anger and resentment to be emotional risk factors for cancer. The weight they carry will vary from person to person.

This is not to blame the patient. The resentment is often buried in the subconscious along with the memories of the event that caused it. Sometimes it can be very hard to heal from our wounds, whether it is the grief of losing a child, feeling betrayed by a spouse or a parent or generalized resentment with life. With time we numb ourselves to the pain, and though it may seem as though we have moved on, the experience leaves a dent in the energy body. The body is very literal when it decides where to store an emotion. For example, witnessing a traumatic event may lead to a loss of sight later in life when a person wishes to un-see the traumatic event. If the experience was a blow to the emotional heart, the memory of the pain can be held in any of the organs that are connected to the Heart Chakra. For example, when life loses its sweetness, that pain may be held in the pancreas. Overwhelm may be felt in the lungs. Or sometimes the dis-ease goes right to the heart itself. In a healing session we send energy to the organ that needs healing and to the emotion that is held there.

As part of the self-healing process, the cancer patient may wish to confront the memory that triggered the emotion. Some will have no trouble identifying the issue. They were hurt and they are conscious of the grudge. They may even feel entitled; after all, some offenses are unforgivable. Others will have buried the memory too deep for recognition, especially if they cannot bring themselves to admit feeling angry or resentful. It is important to be gentle, loving and supportive throughout the process. Self-healing should only peel back layers that we are prepared to deal with. In either case, I would send the energy of love, healing and forgiveness to the tumor without dwelling on why it might be there. If the cancer patient has trouble identifying the issue, sending the mind on a wild goose chase would be counterproductive from a mental relaxation point of view. They may prefer to repeat affirmations for mental and emotional healing. Louise Hay explores this option further in her book: *You Can Heal Your Life*.

As mentioned, each case is unique and I would suggest exploring this theory through meditation and journaling to see if it is relevant.

The following will give you an idea of what to look for, though the list is by no means definitive:

- **Bladder Cancer**. Stifling creativity and abundance with pent-up anger and emotional pain. Anger blocks flow of creative insights.

- **Brain Cancer**. Anger clouds judgment. Cannot see straight or evaluate self objectively.

- **Breast Cancer.** Tendency to over-nurture others and neglect self leads to unconscious resentment. Giving more than receiving. Unable to nurture and care for oneself or others. Nursing a grudge.

- **Cervical Cancer.** Rejecting womanhood. Anger at unequal balance of power in relationships. Low self-esteem.

- **Colon Cancer.** Trouble letting go of past grievances, when even the mind has let go and moved past the experience. Denial.

- **Leukemia**. Holding the belief that life is not beautiful or joyful. Possible past life traumas or "family" memes to heal.

- **Liver Cancer.** Feelings of anger over loss of control. Resent being obliged to live by someone else's rules. Power struggles.

- **Lung Cancer.** Resenting life for repeated blows to the heart. Harboring grief and pain. Depression. Cannot face another day.

- **Lymphoma:** Suppressing our desires, feelings and priorities and instead living according to external expectations of what *should be*.

- **Esophagus Cancer:** A personal truth was swallowed. The body resents being forced to swallow instead of speaking the truth.

- **Ovarian or Womb Cancer**. Feeling disconnected from Goddess Energy. Blocking creative and life-giving force from universe.

- **Pancreatic Cancer.** Resenting life for unfair treatment of someone near and dear to the heart: child, spouse, etc. Feeling hurt or betrayed by a close loved one. Feeling loss of control.

- **Prostate Cancer.** Creativity, passion for life and outward energy stifled. Feeling one has not manifested life purpose and dreams.

- **Stomach and Intestinal Cancer**. Denial and rejection of our truth. Unable to process feelings of anger or resentment.

- **Oral Cancer**. Angry and not speaking truth. Inability to try, taste or swallow life experience. Left with a bitter taste.

If buried anger and resentment are emotional risk factors for cancer, we need to think about forgiveness. This is easier said than done; some offenses are very hard to forgive. Unfortunately, it is the only way to move forward without holding toxic energy in the body. As Buddha said, "Holding onto anger is like grasping a hot coal with the intent to throw it at someone else. You get burned." Forgiveness does not mean condoning a morally reprehensible or unjust action. When we forgive, we wipe all traces of anger and resentment from our energy system. Forgiveness does not happen overnight either; we need time to acknowledge the pain and release it before we can move on. Otherwise forgiving too soon can also have a negative effect on our self-esteem. It takes time to heal.

There is a big difference between forgiving and forgetting. The latter is no better than going into denial about what happened. Though it may be easy enough to function on a daily basis, with time that buried emotion will resurface. Nursing a grudge can be toxic for the person who holds it, whether or not it is justified. The first step is to be aware of the problem. Overcoming the resistance to forgive is the hardest part. When that is done the last step comes naturally. In some cases it may be possible and desirable to seek out a reconciliation with the person involved. The meditations I have included in Appendix 1 are designed to facilitate self-healing through forgiveness, surrender and unconditional love. Even if we have nothing to forgive, they can still help us find peace and comfort in difficult situations.

Note: This hypothesis raises a number of questions that I cannot answer. For example, do anger and resentment always lead to cancer and will healing these emotions also heal the physical body? Though there may be a few instances of spontaneous remission, my intuition tells me that forgiveness will complement medical intervention by clipping the cancer cell's wings, so to speak. Without the energy of anger fueling its growth, the tumor's grasp on the human body can start to fade. It is possible that surrounding the tumor with love and forgiving the offense, whether it was with life, a friend or a family member, will remove that energy from the body and make the cancer cells less resistant to treatment.

Negation of the Self

What about those cancer patients who are sweet as cotton candy, the ones who wouldn't hold a grudge and are quick to let things slide? On the surface, this theory of emotional risk factors would not apply to them. The truth is we all feel the pain of disappointment, but not everyone is comfortable expressing ugly or so-called negative emotions. Though outwardly peaceful, the body is likely to feel and absorb what is not said.

In the second half of the book we will take a close look at the Chakras. Often referred to as Wheels of Light, the Chakras regulate the flow of energy in the body. Ideally, all seven Chakras would be perfectly balanced and our personal energy would flow freely between them. This energy, and the feelings it carries, would be released easily, keeping the physical, mental, emotional and spiritual bodies clear and healthy. The Chakra system is equipped with an outlet that lets us release this energy: the Throat! Speaking the truth and telling people how you feel will empower you and it will also help you release stuck energy. As long as we speak the truth from a loving place (Heart Center), our energy body will be in alignment with our soul purpose. Unfortunately, quite a few people have trouble with this. They might speak their truth in a way that hurts, and we have all been on the receiving side of this disaster at some point in our lives.

Others may not feel entitled to communicate their feelings, especially to family and close friends. This is common in cultures that teach women to be kind, loving, supportive and to some degree submissive. They care for others without asking for anything in return and without speaking up when they need love, attention, care or rest. This brings me back to the case of breast cancer, which I believe to be linked to an imbalanced Heart Chakra. The function of the breasts is to nurture and feed children. If a woman feels obliged to over-nurture others, putting herself second, this puts her at an energetic disadvantage. She might give all her energy away voluntarily, but her body will resent it. In some of my healing sessions, I find the Solar Plexus and Heart Chakras to be at odds with each other. The Heart Chakra's compulsion to give is stronger than the Solar Plexus' self-preservation instincts. These are often repressed because from an early age, we learn to ignore what might be considered selfish instincts.

After some time, this energy imbalance will start to manifest as feelings of sadness, depression or frustration. Those intuitive feelings are the language the body and soul use to tell the conscious mind that something is wrong[7]. It is worth mentioning that this refers to intuitive feelings, not emotions. Emotions are reactions to people or situations. You get mad at someone. You are thrilled to win the lottery. You are frustrated and angry because you did not get the promotion. Intuitive feelings, on the other hand, tend to sweep over us or sit within us without a trigger to explain them. Both will have an impact on our physical and mental health. The intuitive feeling can be harder to decipher. What does it mean if you feel blue on a particular day? Meditation is a good way to tune into these feelings and gain clarity. It is also vital to take the time to do this, because those feelings sit in the physical body until we work through them.

I believe these energy imbalances trigger negative emotions that need to be released if we are to remain healthy. When that does not happen, the body holds those negative emotions, where they become energetic risk factors for disease. The illness we end up getting may depend on the experience that created the emotion. The Heart Chakra enables us to connect with and feel unconditional love. We also bond to the people we love through this Chakra. When that love is shattered, the anger, hurt and pain from the experience may find its way to the organs that are connected to the Heart Chakra. Though the pancreas is usually associated with the Solar Plexus Chakra and control issues, my intuition also points me to the Heart Chakra where cancer is concerned. The pancreas regulates our blood sugar levels through insulin production. Life is not so sweet when we have

---

[7] McLaren, Karla. Your Aura and Your Chakras. San Francisco: Weiser, 1998. Print

been let down by someone we love and trust. The feelings of betrayal, anger and resentment can accumulate in the pancreas. Acknowledging and releasing this emotional burden is part of any healthy self-healing process.

Denying our feelings only leaves them to simmer until they resurface at a later date, whether it is in the physical body or in an emotional outburst that takes everyone by surprise. In the second half of this book we will explore a variety of self-healing techniques to help with this process.

Does any of this mean that illnesses are "our fault?"

Not at all! Blaming ourselves for an illness would be missing the mark. Not to mention the unnecessary stress and pressure for patients. Based on my experience with cancer patients and with support staff in hospitals over the past four years, the belief that 'if cancer is caused by anger, then this is somehow my fault' does a huge disservice to patients.

The idea is to find peace with compassion; self-love and forgiveness while becoming self-aware and modifying behaviors that do not serve us on a personal level. And in the case of striking life events, which any of us would struggle with, we need more awareness of the emotional, mental and potentially physical implications that difficult circumstances bring. If anything, we need to learn to work with our emotions on a daily basis so that our lives are empowered by our changing mood states and not held hostage by them. Karla McLaren has a wonderful book on the subject, called *The Language of Emotions: What Your Feelings Are Trying To Tell You.*

Chapter 2

What Can We Learn by Being Sick?

Making sense of hardships falls into the realm of spirituality rather than science. It is human nature to ask "Why did this happen to me?" Though there may be medical explanations for illnesses, a scientific answer will not help us make sense of the pain and suffering that comes with these experiences. At these moments, many people have traditionally turned to God or to a Higher Power for answers. One of my history teachers in high school hinted at the correlation between tough economic times and the fervor with which cultures believe in a Higher Power. When things go well, we are less likely to look for answers. When things go poorly, we ask why, and we want to find hope that things will get better. Hope and faith are not the answer for everyone. Some find it easier to throw the idea of a Higher Power out the window. We all cope in different ways.

In the previous chapter, I considered a variety of answers to the question "Why do people get sick?" In this section, I will take it one step further, looking at illness from a soul path point of view. These theories are based on a belief in reincarnation, karma and soul purpose. I believe we all come to earth with a purpose and life mission. How and when we choose to leave this life will depend on our ability to deal with challenges. For some, a cancer diagnosis will be a wake-up call. For others it may be that their journey is coming to an end and it is time to make peace with life and with their loved ones before they move on.

The following are a list of spiritual insights and benefits that can be gained from an illness. Some of these might answer "Why has this happened?"

Reinforcing and Redefining Roles in The Family

Let's start with a question: Has the family dynamic changed with the diagnosis? We have already discussed the possibility that a common illness can make us feel connected to a relative who had it in the past. What if we go one step further and think about how the illness can bring a family together? In my dad's case, I would have to admit that we saw a lot more of him after he fell ill. His work involved weekly business trips and those stopped when he could no longer keep up the pace. It is possible that the illness served the life purpose of slowing him down?

The reverse can also be true. When we fell ill as children, our parents took care of us. We would be pampered for a day – the center of attention. Being sick does not feel good but feeling loved does. The mind may mistake that "illness" for a positive outcome because we get the attention we seek. If the patient were to heal, would they miss this? Take a moment to think about what the illness brings your family in terms of closeness and unity. Is there a way to maintain that closeness? Bringing this into the family consciousness may facilitate the healing.

The last scenario involves role reversals. Simply put, falling ill will force a person to accept help and care from others. This can be difficult for an independent person. Sometimes we give too much and we need to take turns receiving to stay balanced. When it comes to healing, balance is key, and that means receiving as much as you give. Though this will be a tough lesson for some, it is also a chance for their loved ones to show their affection and care. This experience will balance out the scales, though admittedly, the learning process is not a pleasant one.

Pressing The "Pause Button"

The human body needs a break. So do the mind, the intellect and the spirit. Life is becoming increasingly fast-paced. Most of us do not take enough time out and our hectic lifestyles can wear the body down. We also lose sight of the things that matter and we end up on autopilot instead of planning our life. I usually get the flu when it is least convenient to take a break. It might be a high-pressure week at work. Being floored by a horrible cold forces me to rest and contemplate on my life. Am I driving myself into the ground with too much stress? Is all my hard work doing anything for my life purpose? Am I happy? When I get sick, it is likely I have not listened to my body's cries for rest. My body takes revenge by knocking me out with a bad cold, with conjunctivitis or with a "bad back."

In the case of cancer, the message would have to be pretty damn significant in the overall scheme of things. In my dad's case, it may have been a wake-up call, telling him he had a family to spend time with instead of traveling five days a week on business. His brain tumor put a dent in his stride, and looking back on it, we might not have seen much of him without the illness. Though I do think the falling out with my granddad was a big factor in his illness, the cancer diagnosis meant he was not able to keep up the pace at work and his priorities changed.

Why someone gets sick is not something I can make sense of but I have considered the possibilities. I would encourage everyone, healthy or not, to have an honest look at their life and think about what they would change if they could start over. This can be enough to get started on the path of self-healing.

A Spiritual Wake-Up Call

I like to think of our time on earth as a personal development plan that the soul agrees to. Caroline Myss has written extensively about a theory of soul contracts that we enter into prior to birth. We start with a learning objective as well as a purpose that we need to fulfill. The learning objectives are a list of lessons we need to learn as we grow up. They can include self-respect, standing up for ourselves, socializing, opening up to love, etc. All of these lessons make us stronger, more well-rounded people. The soul purpose, on the other hand, is about what we bring to this planet. How can we help others? Some people, like Mother Teresa did, find their soul purpose and live it out in the open. Others are more discreet. Still others have trouble identifying any purpose at all. Think about your passions and how you can use them to channel light into the world. Your purpose might be to uphold justice, to lobby for a specific cause, or even to make people laugh. There are lots of issues to champion and lots of ways to get involved. Our purpose is a game changer for the people we touch.

Life has no classrooms, so this learning plan manifests through the people we meet. In my case, I had to learn to deal with strong-willed and controlling authority figures. I have experienced controlling people from an early age. When I went to work I started running into managers who were also controlling. I worried about whether or not they approved of me and I thought the only way get that approval was to do as they said. My voice did not exist in that equation. My bosses got progressively stronger and more outspoken. A few weeks into a new job as a marketing assistant, my boss had me scrambling over the desk to answer the phone when he rang. I did my best to get the job done but nothing seemed good enough. One of my friends gave me a psychic reading and brought this up spontaneously. She mentioned my new boss and then linked it all the way back to my childhood. According to her reading, I kept failing the test, which was "standing up for myself" and "not seeking approval." Quitting was not an option. I had to learn my lesson. Otherwise, I would fall into the same trap.

That day I resolved to change my behavior. As I grew more confident, our relationship improved dramatically. I wound up loving the job and was genuinely sad to go when I was promoted to a new job six months later. Having that self-awareness enabled me to learn the lesson and move on quickly. If we miss the signs, however, the soul will catch our attention with an emergency lesson. A serious illness can do this job, as is the case with any significant wake-up call. If we still have not learned our lesson, the soul might make an executive decision to end this life early so that we can re-group before starting over with a new life. This theory is based on reincarnation, and the concept of the spirit world as a place where we go to rest and to plan our next life. There is an excellent book called *Journey of Souls* by Michael Newton, who goes into this in more detail.

Connecting With Your Life Purpose

The easiest way to explain this is to tell you about my first experience with healing, as a client. When I was 25, I boarded a flight from Egypt to Mexico. It was after a holiday in extremely hot weather (45-50C) and I was dehydrated. The flight flew through Paris on the way back to Latin America and I slept through the last eight hours of the trip. When we finally landed, I had trouble walking because of cramps in my legs. The next day I went shopping with my cousins and we spent about two hours roaming one of Mexico City's shopping malls. By the end of the day my legs were killing me. It was as though I had pulled a muscle. The cramps got worse and after a few days I was limping. I went to see a doctor. By then, I could barely walk, though my legs looked normal. He confirmed that I had a pulled muscle and recommended bed rest and physical therapy. After three trips to the physiotherapist, I was not getting better. She told me it might be my veins. Go see another doctor! As it turned out, I had deep vein thrombosis.

I had been home for three weeks, doing all of the things you are not supposed to do when you have DVT (bed rest, massages, etc.). The clot was about 50 centimeters long when the doctors finally caught it. I should have spent the past few weeks in the hospital. My mom almost fainted when she heard the news. I still cringe when I think back to the massages I had to relieve the pulled muscle. The doctor said I was extremely lucky; I made it through the critical moments with no real care or intervention and I somehow managed to escape without a pulmonary embolism, a heart attack or a stroke. The danger came and went before I knew it. Two days later I was on blood thinners. It took nearly a year for the clot to dissolve.

This experience changed my life in two ways. The most obvious is the realization that I am lucky to be alive. We all are. A few weeks after it happened I went to see one of my college professors who had just been diagnosed with breast cancer. She had gone through surgery and chemotherapy. We got around to talking and I mentioned my recent medical mishaps. I was not fishing for sympathy, just sharing my experience. Her response took me by surprise:

"That could have killed you Regina. God must have big plans for you."

That was the first realization. The second was more of a hassle: I had a history of blood clots! I was also having irregular periods, horrible cramps, and my doctor could not prescribe anything because the standard hormonal treatments are contraindicated for women with history of blood clots. So I started taking Advil and other painkillers in strong doses. Then one day my mom recommended a crystal healer in Mexico City. I remember thinking she had to be crazy. How was a crystal healer going to regulate my hormones and cure my period pains? But then again, how could it leave me worse off? I decided to give it a chance.

I found it hard not to laugh at the first session. She had me lie on a couch and put what felt like pebbles all over me. Over the course of 30 minutes she would take crystals from bowls on a nearby table, put them on my head, shoulders, neck, hips, knees, etc, and then flick her hands in the air. Sometimes she rubbed my shoulders and snapped her fingers. Was she a witch? Or just plain crazy? Back then I was not the least bit spiritual, intuitive or even open to anything the rational mind could not explain. I peppered her with questions about what she was doing, how it worked and what she could sense. She was using the crystals and her intuition to get a feel for my energy. Some of the crystals found their way into a homeopathic remedy. The session cost 20 dollars. The homeopathic remedy about 150. My cramps stopped after a few months and then we moved on to emotional and mental aspects that I wanted to work on. By then, I was sold on crystal healing. She was the first medical intuitive I ever met, though she did not describe herself that way. She was a seer, *vidente* in Spanish.

At this point I was still recovering from the DVT and making monthly trips to the hospital to have an ultrasound on my veins. For four months, I saw the crystal healer and continued with my medical treatment for the clot. Every month the healer would have a look at my leg, telling me the energy was still blocked. She told me I still needed the medication and that the doctors were not likely to take me off it. Then one day, she told me the energy block had gone and she thought the clot was on its way out. I went to the hospital the following week for an ultrasound. The clot was not entirely gone, but it was small enough that the doctor took me off the blood thinners. Hearing it from her, and then from the doctors, made me a believer in healing and psychic abilities.

It was a unique situation because I had simultaneous visits to the healer and to the doctor. The experience tested my skepticism ... and my faith. I do not think that is the reason I had the DVT, but it did move my life in a new direction. Now that I have had a chance to study medical intuition, I am better able to make sense of WHY it happened. In *You Can Heal Your Life*, Louise Hay says the blood is a carrier for joy and life force, which the heart pumps all over the body. I was not happy at the time and I think the joy dried up in my veins. On one level the DVT was a warning sign, yet it also introduced me to healing. I might have found my way eventually but this experience tested my beliefs. Without it, I might not have embraced Energy Healing when opportunity knocked.

Part II
Introduction to Energy Healing

Quantum physics tells us that the universe is made of energy. Everything around us consists of energy, including the human body. Albert Einstein said that "Energy cannot be created or destroyed; it can only be changed from one form to another." This introduction to Energy Healing focuses on our personal energy and how we can transmute it to facilitate the healing process. The concepts I am going to present are based on the Eastern tradition of Chakras and how they relate to our physical, emotional, mental and spiritual health. The Chakras, often referred to as Wheels of Light, regulate the flow of energy in the body. This energy can lift our spirits. But it also can weigh us down when we are stressed. Our thoughts, emotions and feelings have energetic charge. Energy Healing works by clearing stuck and heavy energy, leading to a relaxed and peaceful mood.

The dictionary defines healing as:

1. To make healthy, whole, or sound: restore to health: free from ailment
2. To bring to an end or conclusion, as conflicts between people or groups, usually with the strong implication of restoring former amity…
3. To … cleanse, purify: *to heal the soul*

The first sentence speaks of "restore to health," which can include physical, mental or emotional healing. When faced with a cancer diagnosis, our first thoughts go to the physical body. What is the prognosis? This is the domain of medical intervention. Nevertheless, the diagnosis has a ripple effect on the patient's mental and emotional health. This brings me to the second point: When one person is sick, the whole family suffers. The family also needs to heal from the experience, though their needs may be largely mental and emotional. Finally, the soul can also heal. Each situation is unique; for some people this might be acknowledging their truth. For others it can be unfinished business and grief.

Energy healers channel universal energy, which is readily available to us all. This energy is directed at the Healee's physical, emotional, mental and spiritual body, clearing stuck energy and facilitating the self-healing process. This energy is often visualized as white light. It might go to a specific organ, to a painful memory or it might clear the emotional load on their mind. Clients will typically report feeling mentally and emotionally relaxed after the session. I like to think of Energy Healing as assisted meditation. It can be extremely valuable if you or someone you love is coping with cancer. This book will give you a good understanding of the energy body and how healing can help patients as well their families. It is important, though, to be realistic about what Energy Healing can and cannot do. It should not be expected to eradicate cancer, though it can help in many ways. Here are a few examples:

Benefits for the cancer patient

- Relaxation, stress relief and an emotional outlet.
- Some patients report increased energy levels, making it easier for them to maintain quality of life through chemotherapy treatments.
- Healing can also help terminal cancer patients draw on their inner strength, allowing them to face their fears and move on peacefully.
- The peace and stillness felt during Energy Healing sessions lets their intuition to come through, giving clarity on the challenges faced.
- Energy Healing can also give the patient a fresh perspective on life.

Benefits for the family

- Self-Healing can be used to manage their grief, shock and stress.
- It releases the emotional stress and burden in a healthy and productive way.
- Engaging with self-healing can help family members stay mentally and emotionally clear, which will do a lot for their well-being.
- By learning to give Energy Healing, family members can play an active role in the cancer patient's healing process. This can have a psychological and emotional benefit for the family member, as well as helping the cancer patient in the family. I will describe this in detail, as there are important health and safety considerations for the Healer to follow.

In this book I refer to the person giving the healing as the Healer. This can be a professional energy healer who has been hired by the family or by the patient. But it can also refer to any family members who want to learn to give healing themselves. The person receiving the healing will be referred to as the Healee. This can be the cancer patient as well as family members who wish to receive healing. This book will give you an introduction to the world of Energy Healing. In the reference list at the back I will provide links to schools and online seminars where you can learn more. I hope you enjoy Energy Healing as much as I have. For more information on my sources of inspiration please see the Recommended Reading List in Appendix 4. My understanding of healing has evolved organically with practical case studies, formal training and of course, plenty of reading.

If you have questions I can be contacted on email, Facebook or Twitter:

- Email: geena@diaryofapsychichealer.com
- Facebook Page: www.facebook.com/SelfHealingCancerandLove
- Twitter: @reginachouza

Chapter 3

The Energy Body

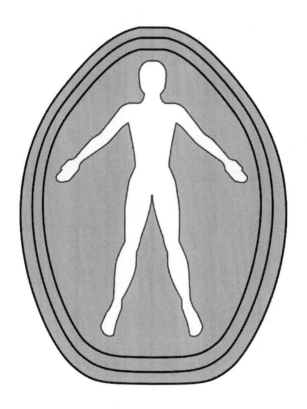

It would be easy to write an entire book on the Chakras and the Aura. For the purposes of this guide, I will cover only the aspects necessary to practice the self-healing techniques in the following chapters. These are designed to be simple enough for beginners to practice. If you have any questions please visit my Self-Healing, Cancer and Love page on Facebook. I will include a list of common questions and answers and will also be available to answer new queries. Over the next few months I hope to bring a group of healers to the page as well. They may have thoughts on dealing with cancer that I have not considered. In time we should have a nice support group for families that are dealing with cancer.

The Aura and The Subtle Energy Bodies

The easiest way to understand the Aura is to imagine a bubble of light around your physical body. It is shaped like an egg and extends above your head, under your feet and out to your sides. This is what we refer to as the human energy field. On any given day, it will extend an arm's length in any direction, though it varies from person to person. If you have ever felt someone walk up behind you, they may have overstepped your auric boundary. The Aura is like a sponge; it absorbs the feelings associated with our day-to-day thoughts and interactions. Clearing the Aura can release tension from the physical, mental and emotional body. Otherwise, these feelings build until we start to feel overburdened. When I am under a lot of stress I try several Aura cleansing techniques, including meditation, breathing exercises, singing or even swimming and brisk walking.

There are as many layers to the Aura as there are Chakras, with estimates ranging from seven to 12. For simplicity, I divide the Aura into four layers:

1. **The physical Aura layer**: This layer is closest to the body. Physical symptoms are often visible in this layer. During a healing session I often scan the Aura with my hands. If I feel heat or tingly sensations close to a particular area, for example the knee, I send healing to this area and then smooth it out with my hands to release the energy. This is done in the auric field without touching the body. After the session I will mention it to the client. If the

42

tingling sensation was in the physical layer, they often comment on a recent bruise, accident or surgery.

2. **The emotional Aura layer**: One of my colleagues asked if a person's Aura changes color with their mood. Indeed it does! The second layer holds our emotional reactions to life. It registers our mood as well as the feelings we absorb from others. An emotional situation generates energetic debris, which can accumulate here. This can affect the way we feel on a daily basis. A daily practice of Aura cleansing can reduce the emotional overload, especially if we are under a lot of stress and tension. Please refer to the Aura Cleansing meditation in Appendix 1 for more information.

3. **The mental Aura layer** holds our thoughts, beliefs, memories and worries. If a person has the tendency to rehash worries over and over again, it will weigh on this layer. Over-analyzing can muddle our thinking capabilities, which is why people like to "get some air" and clear their heads. That practice literally clears the mental Aura layer. Life makes sense when this layer is clear and the answers come to us naturally. I have also found that clients with busy mental layers (especially around the head) tend to complain of headaches. These are linked to repetitive thoughts and worries. Clearing the Aura can help relieve the headache.

4. **The spiritual Aura layer** is linked to the Crown Chakra. Having a strong Crown Chakra gives us clarity, purpose and direction. When that spiritual connection is weak our motivation fades. When the spiritual Aura and the Crown Chakra are clear, we are in tune with our spirit and our life purpose. When it is imbalanced by old and stuck energy, we lose our sense of direction and purpose. It is furthest from the physical body.

The Chakras

The Chakra system is rooted in the Eastern understanding of the human energy field. The Chakras regulate the flow of energy in the human body on a physical, emotional and mental level. The seven major Chakras each relate to a specific area of life, for example: physicality, creativity and passion, self-expression, experience of love, communication, vision and spirituality. When a Chakra is clear and active, that part of life unfolds with ease. We are aligned with the flow of life, ups and downs are easier to navigate. This alignment can be facilitated by a daily practice of meditation and Chakra balancing. For example, think of the last time you had a misunderstanding with a friend. The experience may have left you with an unpleasant aftertaste. That feeling corresponds to an imprint in your Aura, which serves as a reminder and an imbalance. This is what I refer to as energetic debris. It is generated by daily interactions, thoughts and feelings.

Over time, this energetic debris will accumulate until it clouds the Chakras and reduces the flow of energy. This is often referred to as a block, though imbalance is a more appropriate word. Chakras are rarely fully blocked. When a Chakra is out of balance, we start to feel stuck physically and emotionally. By clearing the Chakras we rid ourselves of that feeling and we also re-establish the flow of energy in the body. I like to think of the Chakras as the body's natural air conditioning system. When they are clear and connected, energy flows smoothly and freely. For example, a slow Sacral Chakra may diminish our experience of wealth. It becomes increasingly difficult to *make ends meet*. The challenge may be felt in any of the areas that are typically linked to the Sacral Chakra. If the energy in the body slows down then we may feel aches and pains in a particular organ.

The Chakras are relevant because they regulate the flow of universal energy to the body's many organs and tissues. Each organ is dependent on at least one Chakra, and we can send it healing through that Chakra. When I started studying Energy Healing I noticed that most of my physical complaints were related to the Sacral Chakra: chronic lower back pain, pre-menstrual syndrome, and hormonal imbalances. This is also where I am most often blocked in my life: manifesting wealth, passion, creativity and self-expression. When I give myself healing, I focus on the Sacral Chakra because it directs healing to the places where I need it most, physical or not.

Earlier I introduced the idea of emotional risk factors for cancer, including anger and resentment. It is possible to send healing to these feelings through the Chakra system. For example, if a client were dealing with pancreatic cancer, I would send healing to the Heart Chakra, the pancreas and to the memory that holds that emotional pain. Healing relies on intent, so we only need to hold the Healee's hand to send the energy in that direction. As long as the Healee accepts the healing energy and is willing to release past hurts, that is enough. If the Healer has a qualification in counseling it may be helpful to discuss it. This is not necessary though; merely sending healing to the memory will do. Healing is a gradual process. We may see an effect on mental and emotional health before there are any changes on the physical level. A simple Chakra meditation can clear slow energy from the mental and emotional body.

The major Chakras can be found at the base of the spine, the navel, below the ribs, the heart, the throat, the forehead and on the crown of the head, as follows:

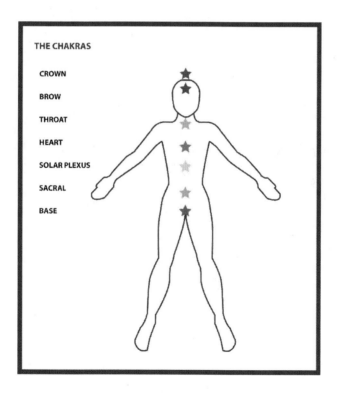

THE CHAKRAS

CROWN

BROW

THROAT

HEART

SOLAR PLEXUS

SACRAL

BASE

There are seven major Chakras:

- The Crown Chakra is our connection to Spirit, God and universal energy. When it activates, you may feel a prickly sensation on your scalp. It is linked to intuition, spirituality and inner knowing. It is often perceived as a soft violet color. Related organs: brain, head, muscles, skeleton and skin.

- The Brow Chakra is linked to the mind, vision, thought and analytical capabilities. It is located at the forehead and may be perceived as indigo in color. Excessive worrying will cloud the Brow Chakra, impairing our ability to see our life clearly and objectively. Related organs: brain, eyes, and nervous system.

- The Throat Chakra is sky blue in color. It rules our communication and self-expression, including listening, speaking and writing. A well-developed Throat Chakra can also help you connect to your intuition, your angels and your soul. If we are holding onto anger or resentment because we have not been able to voice our feelings, sending healing to the Throat Chakra can help. The first step is to accept your truth. The second is to speak it with love and compassion. Related organs: ears, mouth, throat, neck, shoulders, thyroid and esophagus.

- The Heart Chakra is our center of love, both romantic and unconditional. A healthy Heart Chakra will enable you to feel loved, supported and cared for. It is possible to send love and healing anywhere in the body through the Heart; for example sending healing to a tumor through the Heart. Hold the intent of sending the healing light to the rest of the body and visualize the tumor dissolving. This Chakra is often perceived as green or pink in color. Related organs: heart, cardiovascular system, blood, lungs, immune system and the breasts.

- The Solar Plexus is often identified as the seat of the Ego (sense of self), though it also holds the personality. Both should be cared for and stimulated, rather than repressed. It is also the seat of nervousness, anxiety and the body's warning system. The Solar Plexus's "warning system" can go into overdrive when we are under a lot of stress, creating a permanent feeling of uncertainty, anxiety and fear. This can be cleared and healed by sending love and light to the Solar Plexus. It is often seen as bright yellow. Organs: stomach, liver, pancreas, spleen and the digestive system.

- The Sacral Chakra is linked to our creative drive and passion for living. It is connected to the emotional Aura layer and is also the Chakra through which we have energetic exchanges with other people. Clearing the Sacral Chakra can help us release stuck emotions and to heal the emotional Aura layer. This Chakra is relevant for healing ovarian and cervical cancer, as it relates to sexuality, to the ability to give birth to new ideas and creative projects and to fertility. Energy Healing can also be directed to any emotional disappointments in these areas, facilitating emotional healing. The Sacral Chakra is seen as orange in color. Related organs: bladder, colon, hips, kidneys, prostate, ovaries and womb.

- The Root Chakra is linked to community, safety, grounding and feelings of economic and material stability. It is located at the base of the spine. Energy flows from this Chakra into the physical Aura layer, connecting it to the entire body. During a healing session I will often hold one hand over the Root Chakra and the other over the area that needs physical healing. The intent is to clear any imbalances on the physical level. It is usually bright red. Related organs: legs, feet, skeleton, prostate, bowels, lower intestine.

The Aura, the Chakras and the physical body are connected so it is a good idea to include all three in a healing session. Most healers work intuitively and each session will be slightly different. If the client has a physical disease, I will also spend some time with my hands near the affected area. For example, if they have lung cancer I might send healing to the lungs, the Heart Chakra and the cardiovascular system. The breath facilitates the oxygen exchange in the blood, which sends energy to all of the living tissues in the body. Visualization helps us direct the energy. In this case, it might help to visualize the healing energy as white light and imagine it flowing through the entire body including the lungs, heart, blood and the tumor. The Healer and the Healee might also visualize pink light (or another color), if that helps the Healee feel secure during the session.

Chapter 4

Self-Healing Techniques

"Energy Follows Thought" – I first heard this at a class that focused on the energetic bonds we form with loved ones (and with not-so-loved ones). The theory is that all of our thoughts, emotions and feelings are stored as energy. Hanging onto emotions, doubt, worry and stress create clutter in the Aura and eventually in the physical body. More often than not, our negative emotions are directed at the people who triggered the response and we send that energy their way. Loving thoughts are charged with positive healing energy. Fearful thoughts are charged with stress and worry. Angry thoughts leave the thinker agitated. Hanging onto the energy of fear, guilt and resentment can have a strong impact on our well-being. This does not mean we should suppress these feelings. The idea is to acknowledge them and release them in a safe and loving manner.

This notion that we can influence energy with our thoughts is referred to as intent. The key pillars of Energy Healing are intent, trust and connecting to universal energy. Before a healing session I start by specifying that I wish to connect to the purest energy available, that of unconditional love, and I trust it will happen. Unconditional love goes beyond our prejudices and insecurities to loving even those corners that we are ashamed of. Bringing that energy into your being can have a profoundly healing effect on many levels. I like to visualize that energy as white, pink or gold light and visualize it healing the body. It is also possible to give it a specific task; for example: surrounding a cancer tumor with the energy of unconditional love and using your mind's eye to visualize it dissolving the tumor. As such, I use a mix of intent and visualization in all of my sessions. Energy Healing is a very simple process and self-healing can be very powerful as well! With a little intent and a lot of trust, we all can do it. I find it helps if we suspend our disbelief for just 15 minutes each day to self-heal.

Now, on to the good stuff...

Healing with the Heart

The heart's capacity for love may be the most powerful healing tool at our disposal. Love heals fear, anger, anguish and other unpleasant emotions. It can also revitalize the spirit. I am not referring to romantic or familiar love, which is loving someone because of who they are to us. Instead, it is universal love and appreciation. Recognizing and cherishing that spark of light in yourself and others. Some people find it easiest to describe the concept of universal love in religious terms, telling us that God, Jesus or Allah are about unconditional love – and wouldn't it be nice if everyone lived their religion that way. We wouldn't have separation, judgment, discrimination, blame or guilt. Healing these qualities, as well as anger and resentment, is precisely what we need to find peace and harmony.

On a personal level, Heart Chakra meditations can be profoundly healing. I like to imagine a soft violet flame filling my Heart Chakra with warmth. The flame transmutes the energy in my Heart to unconditional love, filling it with warmth until it overflows into the rest of my Chakras. I then use my imagination to see and feel it filling every last cell in my body, until I can see myself as love. If I run into resistance, in the form of fear, pain or anxiety, the violet flame releases it too. This also enables me to extend that violet flame to any people or situations around me who need it. To do this, I visualize a similar violet flame filling their Heart Chakras. From this place of love it is easier to handle any personal issues that resurface during self-healing. We merely observe them from a place of love.

Focusing our mind and heart on love can also help us release any pain from the past, especially any memories or experiences that might be linked to the cancer journey. This can be used to help you clear, heal and release any beliefs about cancer that may hold back the healing process. It is also a lovely way to release the emotional burden in the home, as children and pets can be especially sensitive. It is important, however, to see and feel ourselves as unconditional love before extending the violet flame to others or to the home. This releases any fears or worries, replacing them with love.

Talk to Your Body

I enjoy yoga and stretching exercises because they prompt me to listen to my body. When I first tried yoga I noticed tension in my muscles, especially around the neck and shoulder area. This prompted me to start relaxing on a daily basis. It also reminds me to breathe and be more in tune with my body and how it feels. Paying attention to our body's messages is important and we should all do it. But even this is only half the battle. Communication is a two-way street, and we need to consciously give and receive messages. That little voice in your head that says "I am too dumb," "too fat," "too slow" or "getting old" sends messages to the body and the psyche. My teachers call it "noise pollution" and we could all do without it.

Instead, talk to yourself with kindness and watch for any responses. The body can be very communicative with intuitive thoughts and feelings. But it can also be confused, tired and upset. One dimension of Energy Healing is listening to the signs and responding with care. This is often referred to as medical intuition: tuning to the body and letting it show its feelings and emotions. The only thing you need to do is tap into your imagination, your subconscious and your body.

Medical intuition is based on the following:

The human body stores emotions in our organs, our soft tissues, our bones, our glands, our blood etc. They are also held in the subtle energy body, which makes up the Aura. As an intuitive healer, I may notice these things when I scan a Healee's physical body. For example, on several occasions I have found anger or resentment in a Healee's pancreas. More often than not, the feeling is directed at someone close to the heart. It could be a parent, who we would expect love from unconditionally. They might also be disappointed because of a turn of events that seemed brutally unfair.

51

The organs also store emotions and they will let us know how they feel. Try the Color Healing Meditation below to visualize the emotions and the tumor dissolving. I would suggest doing the guided meditations with a friend or a healer, so that they can comfort and guide the Healee through the process. The role of the Healer is to hold the space and help their Healee feel secure and safe. Some of the healing meditations may be emotional to follow, and having a Healer nearby for support and guidance can help, whether it is a professional healer or a family member who acts in that capacity.

My dad was on radiation therapy after his first surgery. It was not a great experience, but he was lucky enough not to go through chemotherapy. The mind and the body have breaking points. I think this is where Energy Healing plays the greatest role: soothing and releasing tension. This can be done with a simple meditation, no longer than 15 minutes, by following these simple steps:

1. Sit or lie down, and visualize a soft white light enveloping the entire body. Use your inner voice to reassure and comfort your body.

2. Then take a few minutes to explain the healing process to the body, including any medical interventions that are planned.

3. Now turn your attention to the T-cells, the body's antibodies, thank them for defending your health and ask them to keep up the good work as the treatment continues. Send them love and strength to carry on.

The body absorbs many signals from the mind, including our choice of words. Never refer to an illness as "my illness." The word "my" implies that you own it. The body thinks it needs to look after it. Instead, use "the illness" or "the cancer."

Though it may be hard to accept, tumor cells need more love, forgiveness and compassion than the rest of the body. In my mind, I see the tumor as a dark reddish-brown energy that holds on fiercely and is afraid to let go. What we want to do is soothe, relax, and encourage the tumor to give up. Rather than ignore the tumor, send it light and tell it to go: kindly, firmly and resolutely. This is where the color healing meditation works well, as the Healee can assign a color to the tumor, interpreting the emotion and significance by its appearance. Shedding light on the underlying issue will help with mental and emotional healing.

Color Healing and Visualization

One of my favorite healing techniques involves visualizing colorful energy in the body and the Aura. I sit in a quiet place and use my mind's eye to scan for any energy that feels out of place, slow or tense. When I find an area that I want to work on, I use my imagination to give it a color. This makes it easier to identify the emotion that is held in that part of the body. For example, if I see or feel the color blue in my shoulder it could represent an undercurrent of sadness. The healing involves asking what this blue represents. The subconscious answers the question with an intuitive thought or feeling. The location in the body can also give clues. For example: The sadness might be in my shoulder because I did not reach out for help. We can work on releasing the color with a simple meditation.

Color Healing Meditations involve bringing your attention to the color and letting yourself feel it. Because the meditation is done with the intent to heal, merely directing your attention to the color will bring the consciousness of healing to that part of your body. You may start to notice intuitive thoughts, emotions and feelings. Memories might also surface and this is part of the process. It helps to observe the feelings, bless them with love and let them go. When that is done, bring your attention back to the color and visualize it filling with white or pink light. The light dissolves the color and releases the emotion from the body so that your personal energy can flow freely again. The meditation can be used on any part of the body, the Chakras or the Aura. It can also be used to visualize the tumor as a color and dissolve the emotional energy it holds.

It is worth noting that the same color can represent different things to different people. For example, grey often signals apathy to me. If I notice grey in a Healee's Solar Plexus I would take it to mean they are apathetic about taking control of their life, as the Solar Plexus is the personal power center. For others it might represent the qualities of iron. They might sense grey energy in their Healee's Solar Plexus and take it to mean that they are extremely strong. The person who sees the color relies on their intuition to interpret it. Colors are not inherently good or bad, they are just signals from the subconscious. No matter what color we see or feel, it can be healed and released using the same guided meditation. It is important that we embrace whatever we find, even if it makes us feel uncomfortable. Fill it with light and let the power of love heal it.

Journaling

Writing is an effective way to release pent-up stress and emotions, especially if we do not want to unleash these feelings on others. Writing can be private, though some people also like to share their thoughts on an online blog. By writing we connect with our emotions and release them from the body and the mind. It is also a great way to channel your sense of inner knowing. There is a technique called Automatic Writing that can be used to let your angels speak through you. I also ask my angels to channel healing through me while I write.

It is a very simple technique:

1. Ground Yourself. Bring your attention to the soles of your feet, your chair and the ground underneath you. Feel the weight of your body and make sure you are fully grounded in the room. Let go of stress so that it drops from your body, through the floor, to the center of the earth where it is absorbed and cleansed.

2. Ask for Protection. Visualize yourself in a bubble of soft protective light. Any color will do, though white and pale pink and blue seem to be most popular.

3. Open Up. Close your eyes and visualize the Universe expanding in every direction. The North Star shines over you. Use your intent to connect to its star energy and watch as it sends rays of light in your direction. I prefer white light for guidance and protection.

Now here comes the fun part – pick up a pen and paper!

4. Tell us what's on your mind! Pour your heart out. Write a full page with all of the things that are bogging you down. This clears the air and creates a space for healing and clarity to come through in the writing. The energy of your emotions should start to shift in a positive direction as you release any baggage and start to focus on your inner self.

5. Pay Attention. There comes a moment when the mind chatter fades and the tone of voice changes. The words you are writing start to calm you down, and the messages are reassuring and peaceful. This is when your angels start to come through; in my case the narrative will often change from the first to the second person.

6. Trust What's Coming to You. One of the things I struggle with is where the info comes from. Just go with the flow and let it out. Use this as an outlet for your stress, feelings and emotions. It is not always necessary to read what you have written afterwards, especially if you are voicing your fears. I like to imagine that all my worries are poured out, and the angels take them from me. This technique can help you let go and to heal at the same time.

Laughter

We have a term back home called *Risoterapia*. It is based on the Spanish words for laughter (*risa*) and therapy (*terapia*). Laughter brings the healing energy of joy into the body. When we laugh the diaphragm starts moving in funny ways, the breath catches and the oxygen exchange in the lungs is altered. The energy of joy and laughter enters the bloodstream through the lungs; it travels to the heart, which then pumps joy all over the body. Laughter is also a muscle and mood relaxant. Joy has strong healing qualities, so watch a funny movie, listen to jokes and laugh your heart out. I have no scientific proof for this whatsoever; call it a hunch.

Soul Healing and Reconciliation

Earlier I discussed the possibility that anger and resentment are risk factors for cancer and that we can heal the emotional scars by forgiving those involved. In some cases it will also be helpful to speak to the person from the heart, airing our grievances in a loving manner and expressing our desire for a reconciliation. If we are unable to speak to them for whatever reason – for example, they may have passed away or might not be receptive to dialogue, we can speak to their soul instead. There are several ways to go about this:

- Start with the Heart Healing meditation and then write a letter to the person telling them how you feel, what their relationship means (or meant) to you. Explain your feelings from a place of love and try to see things from their point of view as well. Send them love and bless their soul with peace.

- Imagine yourself having a heart to heart with the person. This is safe as you are both protected by a violet flame which transmutes negative energy to love. Tell them how you feel and express your desire to reconcile once and for all. Listen to how they feel, trusting your intuition to speak honestly and lovingly on their behalf. Ask for a sign of peace, perhaps a white dove, and let it fly to their soul with this message.

By engaging on a soul level we allow both sides to heal and move on. This will also enable us to relieve any trace of mixed feelings such as guilt, grief or blame which can hold back our own healing process.

Fruits and Vegetables

As I am writing this, my intuition is whispering the word WATER. We get water from fruits and vegetables. We can also get it from bottled water, so drink up! My area of interest is Energy Healing, not nutrition, so please seek professional advice, but I believe eating fresh, leafy greens and drinking plenty of water will facilitate the body's natural healing process.

Please consult your doctor before making any changes to your diet. Some foods have been known to interfere with certain cancer drugs. Though it may seem like a good idea to eat plenty of citrus fruits, only your doctor can advise on what is appropriate for you. The MacMillan Cancer Support website also has general advice for people living with cancer.

Listening to Music

Music can be liberating. It also gives us a chance to work through feelings that we would not know how to voice. Music can soothe us; it can lower our mood and then raise it again with an upbeat tempo. The lyrics can voice thoughts that we are not ready to speak of, allowing us to acknowledge deep emotions. The key here is to let it out, go with the music and let your spirit find a release. Starting with a few sad songs is great as long as we end on a peaceful note that boosts our state of mind. The heart will also find peace and comfort in the music listened to.

Meditation

This is one of my favorite healing techniques. It can be as simple as focusing on your breath for a few minutes and letting your worries slip away. I like to sit under a tree and listen to the wind. It is also possible to meditate on a particular Chakra, visualize it clearing and use your intent to release tension and stress. Appendix 1 contains a series of meditations that can be used to channel love and healing to the body, the Aura and the Chakras. These meditations can be broken down into an opening sequence, the core visualization and the closing.

They each serve a purpose:

1. Opening. The first few phrases are designed to quiet the Healee's mind, and help them connect to the natural rhythm of their breath.

2. Core. The visualization directs the healing energy of Love through the body and in some cases to the cancer cells. I have presented a variety of meditations, including light, color and feeling. Please have a read through these and try the ones that feel comfortable.

3. Closing. The last lines of the meditation are designed to bring your consciousness back into the room. I have ended most of these by prompting you to bring your attention back to your breath and to the weight of the chair under your body. Without this step, you may feel ungrounded or dizzy when the meditation is over. If at any moment you feel lightheaded, stop the meditation and bring your attention to your feet and to the chair under you.

It is usually easier to follow visualizations when someone guides us through the process. For this reason, I would suggest doing these in groups or with a friend. I have also included a few guided meditations on the Self-Healing and Cancer page on my blog and on my YouTube channel, below:

- www.diaryofapsychichealer.com/p/healing-cancer-with-love.html

- www.youtube.com/c/ReginaChouza

Chapter 5

What Do Energy Healers Do?

Energy healers are channels for universal energy. This energy is channeled into the Healee's physical and energy body, where it can balance and reestablish the flow of energy. The energy enters the Healer's body through the Crown Chakra (top of head) and flows through the heart, the arms and out the palms. In a contact healing session, the Healer will stand in the client's auric field. They may start by placing their hands on the client's shoulder and tuning into their energy. At this point, I usually allow the energy to flow gently through the client's body to the ground. My intention is to help them relax before the session starts. I would then move on to clear the Chakras and the Aura. The session may include light touch, with permission from the client. If the client is in a hospital or a small room, it may be easier to sit and hold hands. The energy goes where it is needed and the Healer can also use their intent to send it to a specific area in the body.

Energy Healing sessions can be silent, with the Healer channeling the energy and visualizing its movement through the body. They can also be interactive, with the Healer guiding the client through a meditation while channeling energy. I have included a number of meditations in the first appendix. They are all based on the healing techniques that I learned as part of the course work in healing school. For example, I included a White Light Meditation that involves visualizing the tumor contained in white light and intending for that light to dissolve its energy. These visualizations help release anger, hurt and resentment from the physical body. They can be done alone or with a friend. I have also linked to several Guided Meditations from the Self-Healing, Cancer and Love page on my blog.

What is the difference between Energy Healing and Reiki?

Reiki is a Japanese Energy Healing technique for stress reduction and relaxation that also promotes healing on the physical, emotional, mental and spiritual levels. Having its roots in a Buddhist approach to spirituality and personal development, Reiki relies on universal spiritual energy, which is channeled through the Healer to the Healee. It facilitates the client's self-healing, with less intent and direction by the Healer. Because Reiki is intelligent energy, it goes where it is needed and the client only has to accept it. The quantity channeled will also adjust to the Healee's needs. At a conceptual level this is slightly different to Energy Healing, where the Healer plays an active role directing the energy through the body. Based on my experience with both Reiki and Energy Healing, they do have different vibrations, which I can only describe as different flavors of healing energy. All energy comes from the same place and I believe the end result is the same. Reiki is well known, which has its advantages.

Reiki Practitioners and Teachers are fairly accessible in the US and Europe, making it easy to book a session or to learn Reiki yourself. Reiki is taught through a series of weekend workshops that include theory, hand positions and more importantly, an attunement to Reiki. The word Reiki can be translated as *Rei* = divine intelligence, and *Ki* = life force energy. We already have life force energy (Ki) flowing through our body. The Reiki attunement brings divine intelligence into the equation. The Reiki I attunement allows us to channel energy through the palms of our hands. It also initiates a cleansing process in the newly attuned Healer and for three weeks after we are advised to give ourselves daily self-treatments, get plenty of rest and eat healthful foods. Once the adjustment period has passed, we are able to give Reiki to family and friends. Self-healing with Reiki can be useful for healthy family members who also need to care for themselves. Once they have learned to give healing without depleting their own energy, they can use Reiki to give each other healing, including the cancer patient in the family. All of this can be done with a Reiki I attunement.

The next level of Reiki training involves a second attunement where Reiki students learn to direct the healing energy with the use of symbols. These symbols can be used to send healing to the past, to the future, to the root cause of a particular ailment. For example, in my dad's case I would have used the symbols to send Reiki to the place in his body that held the memory of the tension with Abuelo. It is also possible to send Reiki to whatever is triggering the cancer on a biological level. There is also a symbol that focuses on mental and emotional healing. Attending a Reiki II workshop will enable you to tap into the skills used at a professional level, though these are not to be taken lightly. It is important to be attuned to these symbols by a Reiki Master before you try to use them. Otherwise they are said to act as magnets for unwanted energy. With a proper Reiki attunement and training, the symbols are perfectly safe and pleasant to use.

Note: I have been deliberately brief with this introduction because Reiki can only be channeled after a formal attunement has taken place. Please contact a Practitioner to book a session or a Reiki Master if you would like to learn Reiki yourself.

Finding the Right Healer for You

Most people have heard of Reiki. But there are dozens of healing modalities out there. These include Theta Healing, Spiritual Healing, Angelic Reiki, Angelic Healing, Faith Healing, Cellular Healing, and Heart and Soul Healing. On some level, all healers ground and connect to universal energy. As long as the Healer uses her intention to channel healing energy, the label should not matter. The bigger question is, do you trust the individual? With so many Healers available, the choice can be overwhelming. The most important thing is to find a healer you can trust – one who is open, honest and supportive during healing session.

I believe anyone can learn to give healing. All it takes is meditation, practice and a good teacher to guide you through the process. In Chapter 6, titled Energy Healing for The Family, I will take you through an introduction to Hands-on-Healing, including simple steps that you can follow to heal each other at home. This can give the family an active role in the patient's healing process. It also enables the rest of the family to give each other much needed healing.

Nevertheless, there are disadvantages to working with someone you know (such as a family member or a friend) rather than a qualified Healer. If the person channeling the healing is attached to the Healee, they are more likely to become emotionally invested in the healing. This can deplete their energy and cause them to burn out. An exhausted family member will not be able to help. Learning to channel healing without becoming emotionally invested in the outcome is a difficult lesson; one that all Healers need to learn before they start practicing professionally.

Energy healers are taught to be compassionate, professional and objective. This last point is important because we need to channel healing without being attached to an outcome. There may be times when a person will remain ill until they have learned a particular lesson. In these cases, the Healer facilitates the Healee's awakening, relying on their experience and studies. There are schools where Healers learn about the flow of energy in the body, the meaning behind particular symptoms and how it relates to human behavior. Intuition also plays a big role, as each case is unique. Energy healers also follow a practice of daily meditation, cleansing and personal care, which enables them to channel energy consistently. In this way, a professional Healer will be a stronger channel for energy and they will also have training on the psychological, emotional and spiritual aspects discussed earlier. They are also able to distance themselves from the situation, which brings perspective and a renewed sense of energy.

The rates charged for healing sessions vary, ranging from volunteers who give healing for free, to those who charge hundreds of dollars. Regardless of the price, there are a number of criteria to keep in mind when choosing a healer:

1. Does the Healer claim to cure the disease? There is no way an energy healer can guarantee this outcome. Each situation is slightly different and the healing might only work on the emotional or spiritual aspects. Think about what you would expect to gain from the healing. It might be emotional support, a quiet space to reflect and heal or just a convenient Aura cleanse. Healing might also help you face your fears with courage and dignity, by releasing stuck emotions and clearing

anxiety from the Solar Plexus. This is why I would suggest Energy Healing for the entire family. Remember that the Healer merely facilitates your own self-healing process. They do not fix or cure the Healee.

2. Though not all healers go through formal training, there are several schools in Europe and the United States that teach Energy Healing in depth. The UK has an association called the British Alliance of Healers, which ensures accredited healers have two years of supervised schoolwork and case studies. The Barbara Brennan School in Austria trains its students for more than three years. Qualified Healers may also discuss ongoing case studies with more experienced Healers, who advise on different healing techniques. Nevertheless, there are plenty of people with natural healing abilities. Trust your intuition and do not ignore a gifted Healer because he lacks a qualification.

3. Choose someone who makes you feel comfortable and relaxed. Trust your intuition. Most healers will be compassionate, professional and non-judgmental.

4. How much do they charge and what do they offer in return? Healers need to pay their bills, so it is not uncommon to charge. Some hospitals will sponsor Healers, while others will subsidize their sessions. It is also common to find Healers who volunteer during weekends and at free Energy Healing clinics.

Chapter 6

Energy Healing for The Family

Dealing with cancer is rough on the whole family, not just on the person who is sick. I certainly felt it when my dad was ill. The recovery from his surgery was stressful for everyone involved. I was scared, for example, that he might fall down and hurt his head. I also was worried about the future. The loss of control can be numbing, and everyone finds a different way to cope with this stress. Some of us are less constructive than others.

I had just come home from boarding school in Switzerland, where I had packed on the pounds thanks to an un-ending supply of Swiss chocolate bars. Losing the weight seemed like the natural thing to do, and by the time my dad got sick I had already lost 12 pounds. Only three more to go! I got to my normal weight, and kept going. By then I was also going to the gym every day, usually for two hours. Obsessing over my size, shape and exercise regime was a distraction.

After a few months I lost enough weight that I stopped getting my period. That was when I started to miss food. So I started binge eating for a few weeks, then going back on a diet. I kept my weight in the same range through senior year in high school and then at college I let go. I gained 20 pounds freshman year, and lost it over the summer. My weight went up and down for four years. I was the Queen of Crash Diets during the summer holidays and then I would put the weight on again during the school year. Eating quenched my anxiety. I stopped caring about my weight after Dad's third and final tumor appeared. I got on the treadmill one day and realized it did not matter anymore. That day I stopped doing crash diets and I stopped binge eating. The weight came off slowly and it has not been an issue since then. The word "diet" has no place in my vocabulary, though I do try to eat fresh and healthy food whenever possible.

The connection between my weight and Dad's illness only dawned on me recently. I was "cured" of my neurosis when our worst fears had come true. There was nothing to do about it. Slowly things went back to normal, though of course, the situation was anything but normal. Looking back on it, Energy Healing could have helped me in so many ways. The fear, anxiety and loss of control can be managed by sending healing to the Solar Plexus Chakra. My whole family might have benefited from Energy Healing, though not everyone would have been receptive to it. Healing is there for anyone who wants it, but accepting it is a personal choice. There are different ways to cope including journaling, listening to music and laughing. Some of us like to give and receive Energy Healing. (That is the other secret: Giving healing also soothes and heals the Healer!)

In this chapter I will cover the how-to's of Hands-on-Healing so that you can practice healing each other at home. I also would encourage you to sign up for a Reiki I class or an Energy Healing workshop. Channeling is simple, but managing our energy levels takes practice. We need to leave our emotions, fears, and wishes to one side. Otherwise we can burn ourselves out. A good way to avoid this is to call on angelic energy for help. Let the angels heal through you, and focus on holding the space for the Healee during the session.

Healing With The Angels

If you have read my blog, Diary of a Psychic Healer, you may have noticed that I enjoy working with angels. They can be very grounding, loving and supportive. We can ask for help with any kind of healing and they are more than happy to step in. They can fill our hearts with love, forgiveness, and strength. We all have guardian angels at our beckon call. But we can also work with Archangels for deeper emotional healing. Archangel Raphael, in particular, specializes in the healing of children, animals, the earth and also adults. I find his energy to be grounding and comforting, especially on an emotional level. Sometimes it is easy to feel his presence as warmth in the Heart Chakra, a tingle on your face or even a green flash in your mind's eye. He will show up, so sit quietly and wait for his energy to surround you. A regular practice of meditation will make it easier to sense his energy. This can be as simple as observing your breath for a few minutes everyday and letting the world fade into the background.

Many Healers draw on angelic energy during their healing sessions. Raphael can also step in when we are undergoing medical care, even surgery. Sometimes I will call on him if I am going to the dentist or to a doctor's appointment, asking him to guide the dentist's hand, heart and vision during the appointment. When I have family or friends going into surgery I do the same. The goal is to help the medical team be at their sharpest and most intuitive. I trust that Archangel Raphael is there and I let him do his job. The trick is to ask for his help and then hand the problem over to him. At that moment we need to make a conscious decision to trust Raphael and the medical team to take over. Stop worrying and trust that the angels will look after our best interests (which they will always do!), which may be emotional, mental or spiritual healing.

In the next section I will take you through a few simple steps to channel Healing Energy. These are meant to help beginners through the healing process. I have included angelic healing, so that the novice Healer can pass the responsibility for the healing over to Archangel Raphael. This allows the novice Healer to detach from the outcome and act as a channel. In this book I ask Archangel Raphael for help. It is also possible to call on Jesus, Lord Ganesh, Kwan Yin or any other spiritual figure. This is still Energy Healing because the intent is to clear the Aura and the Chakras by channeling energy. If you would prefer to channel healing without involving these spiritual figures, please use your intent to channel pure white, pink or clear light. Set your intent on channeling light of the highest vibration.

How to Channel Healing Energy

The novice Healer starts with a short meditation to prepare for the healing session. She may like to wash her hands or take a deep breath before starting. The novice Healer should initially stand a few feet away and only approach the Healee after completing the following steps:

1. Ground Yourself. Sit down on a comfortable chair. Imagine sitting with your back to a tree trunk. Now visualize roots coming out of the bottom of your feet, sinking down to the very center of the earth. The roots are as thick as the tree's roots; they are solid and provide support for your physical body.

   Visualize a pink quartz stone at the center of the earth that is full of the healing energy of love. The roots wrap around the pink quartz stone and absorb its healing energy. That energy travels up the roots, up your legs, to your heart. Visualize and feel your Heart Chakra as it fills with earth energy. This energy supports the Healer during the session, but is not passed on to the Healee.

2. Attune to The Energy. Now bring your attention to the North Star. Visualize a beam of white light coming out of the sky, from the stars to your Crown Chakra. If this makes you (the Healer) feel light-headed or dizzy, take your attention back to the roots and just let the white light travel from your Crown to your Heart Chakra. This activates your ability to channel energy. If you would like to incorporate angelic energy into the healing, now is the time to call on Archangel Raphael. You can ask him to stand behind you or to add his energy to the white light flowing through your Crown Chakra if that feels more appropriate and comfortable.

3. Ask for Permission. The next step is to ask the Universe for permission to give healing. You might also ask that the Healee receive whatever form of healing she needs. This step allows the Healer to detach from the outcome; it acknowledges that we are merely channels for healing energy.

4.   Ask for Protection. Visualize a bubble of white protective light around your Healee and around yourself. This white light calms, soothes and protects the both of you, keeping any tension, stress or worry away during the healing.

You are now ready to start the healing session. There are two ways to go about it. One is to stand behind the Healee and gently place your hands on her shoulders. For this to work, the Healee would have to sit in a chair with the Healer behind. As a healer you can visualize white healing light entering your Crown Chakra, flowing down your arms and out your hands and into the Healee's body. The second option is to sit beside the Healee and hold her hand. The white light would flow through your hand to her body during the session.

You may prefer to sit quietly and visualize that white light flowing during the entire session. Keep your first sessions short, not more than 5-10 minutes. After a few sessions, the novice Healer may feel confident visualizing the flow of energy in the physical body during the session. Use your imagination to visualize the body healing itself naturally. If the Healee is a family member who does not have cancer, imagine her Aura and Chakras filled with white light. This light is all that is needed to receive the healing and clear their energy. If the Healee is undergoing treatment for cancer, the following visualizations can be used to send healing to the tumor and the body. The Healer uses her intent and imagination to "tell" the energy what to do, while holding the Healee's hand.

The Healer visualizes this silently from start to finish:

1.   Visualize white light flowing out of the palm of your hands into the Healee's body. This white light is full of unconditional love. It also carries the energy of forgiveness and release. These feelings gently fill the Healee's body and soul.

2.   Bring your attention to the tumor and visualize it filling with soft healing light. The light can be white, purple or pink in color; choose a color that represents the quality of love and healing. The

healing light fills the tumor, reaching every last cell. It deactivates the tumor, releasing any anger, resentment or fear.

3.   Through your intent, this white light dissolves the cancer cells and the tumor loses its grasp on the human body. Hold this visual for a few minutes until it fades away.

4.   Stay with these images for as long as it feels appropriate, but not more than 10 minutes. Thank Archangel Raphael for his help with the healing session. Step out of the Healee's Aura and visualize her in a protective bubble of light.

5.   The next step is to disconnect from the healing energy. This can be done by bringing your attention back to the North Star and slowly letting that connection fade. Bring your attention back to your feet, your roots and draw your Aura in around you. The last step is to clear your energy. I like to imagine myself under a waterfall and it washes away all of the excess energy from my Aura. This clears my energy so that I do not hold onto any of the emotional or psychological energy that the Healee releases during the session. Once that is done, visualize yourself in a protective bubble of light and thank the universe for the healing.

6.   It is now time to let the Healee know the session is over. You may like to touch her shoulder gently and wait for her to come around. She may have fallen into a deep sleep, give her as much time as she needs to awaken. It may help to bring her attention to her breath, as this will bring her consciousness back to the room. Well done!

Interactive Healings

When I first began healing I was surprised that people felt the energy during the healing session. Some of my clients even saw flashes of color in their mind's eye if I was working on a particular Chakra. For example, if I gave healing to the Solar Plexus they might see a hint of yellow in their mind's eye. This served as confirmation for both of us, and it also helped them engage with the healing. I find that some people are able to perceive the healing and others are not. Either way, the healing still takes place. If the Healee does not see or feel anything during the session, they may prefer to be guided through a meditation to feel more involved in the healing.

Interactive Healings involve guided meditations and dialogue. The Healer still follows the Grounding, Attuning, Protection and Permission steps. Instead of placing their hands on the Healee's shoulders, they sit with them and guide them through a meditation. I have included several meditations in Appendix 1; they can be used to clear, balance and heal the Chakras, the Aura and the body. If you would like to try an Interactive Healing as a family, sit in a circle and have one person guide the meditation. Begin by visualizing a bubble of light around the group before starting the meditation. My favorite is the Purifying and Relaxing Meditation. It goes through each muscle to release tension. This meditation can help the family clear and balance the emotional and mental tension as a group.

Special Considerations for Novice Healers:

Channeling healing takes practice. It took me two years to get to the point where I could channel healing energy consistently. Most of the time I focus on channeling energy and using intuition to guide my movements during the session. The challenge is learning to give healing without becoming emotionally involved and without "pouring your heart out." When this happens, the Healer often experiences an energetic high, followed by a crash. This is not a pleasant experience, believe me! It can be very hard to stay emotionally detached if we are giving healing to someone we love, especially when they are sick. It might help to approach the healing session with scientific curiosity and just see what happens. Leave it to the angels. This open and curious approach facilitates the healing session, without putting the novice Healer in jeopardy.

It is also important for the novice Healer to take special care with their health. When I attuned to Reiki my energy changed dramatically, and I made an effort to drink lots of water, eat healthy and get lots of sleep. I also gave myself Reiki treatments for 5-10 minutes every day. With all of this, I was still tired and grouchy. Giving healing can bring about a short-term crisis while our body adjusts to these new energetic settings. The family's novice Healers need to keep an eye on this and give each other healing as well as the cancer patient. If you have ever been on a flight, you will have seen the instructions for putting oxygen masks on children. Parents are urged to look after their own oxygen masks before helping their kids. This is a practical consideration; they won't be able to look after their kids if they run out of oxygen first.

I would suggest keeping healing sessions at 5-10 minutes length. It could also be a good idea for different members of the family to give each other healing, so long as they are drawn to it. I would also suggest the entire family engage with some of the techniques in the Self-Healing chapter to release stress and to relax.

Please refer to Appendix 3 for an introduction to energy management. It includes grounding, cleansing and protecting exercises for novice Healers.

Epilogue

Something changed a few weeks after I completed what I thought to be the final draft of this book. It was your typical grey day in London and I woke up early to make the long commute to the Lynda Jackson McMillan Centre at Mount Vernon Hospital. I was there to attend a training day for complementary therapists who volunteer in hospitals with cancer patients. The agenda was a broad introduction to cancer, how it is treated and the challenges often faced by patients. It also gave us an idea of how we could help and what advice we could give patients through the different stages.

Some of the information I was familiar with already, for example that diet and obesity are huge risk factors for cancer – the downside of modern living. The World Health Organization claims that a third of cancer cases can be prevented just by addressing these factors[8]. Other concepts were new to me. I did not know that maintaining a light level of physical activity during radiotherapy treatments helps patients minimize the experience of fatigue, which usually peaks two weeks after treatment has concluded. These and other suggestions are available on the McMillan website.

For me, the cancer statistics were the surprise of the day. The media has done a good job scaring us with sound bytes about genetic risk, what percentage of the population can expect to get cancer, etc. – it makes you wonder where we are headed. They do not tell us that cancer mortality rates

[8] World Health Organization, Cancer Fact Sheet, No 297 - May
http://www.who.int/mediacentre/factsheets/fs297/en/index.html

are actually decreasing: more and more people are *surviving* cancer. Based on my dad's experience, deep down I still believed cancer was not something we bounce back from. This made me realize how important it is to examine our beliefs as they can paint us into a corner. At best, a false belief will lead to unnecessary anxiety, at worst it could become a self-fulfilling prophecy.

The fact is, more and more people are surviving cancer every day. Even the dramatic rise in incidence began to taper off in the late Nineties. Though this does not make the news, it is absolutely brilliant and we can credit these statistics to the breakthroughs in medical care. That day, I was surprised to see how far treatment has come since my dad was diagnosed 15 years ago. Some of the newer treatments read like science fiction: hormone and biological therapies that interact with the body at the cellular level, motion detectors on laser therapies that adjust to the patient's breath and moving diaphragm, etc. The weight given to screening programs also means more patients are diagnosed early, giving them a much better chance of survival.

Despite the big wins, we still have a long way to go. The survival rates for some of the more aggressive cancers have hardly budged. I would like to see Energy Healing and science work together when it comes to research and treatment. Imagine what we could accomplish if oncologists trained in medical intuition. They are not without their spirit guides and angels, though skepticism might make some slightly less aware. Intuition can point us in the right direction so that we find our way quicker. Our angels and guides also give us answers or clues when we are stuck. I often use my intuition at work and it helps me stay ahead of the curve. It might seem far fetched but all we need is a handful of intuitive researchers and doctors.

In the meantime, complementary therapists will continue to look after the patient's emotional wellbeing as well as the family's. It is after all, a human condition. Writing and volunteering are how I chose to do my part with the human side. No one should have to face a cancer diagnosis alone. There are several outreach programs that try to help, though resources are often limited. In the UK we have McMillan Cancer Support as well as smaller cancer support centers that serve their local communities. A great example is the Community Cancer Centre in West London, which offers complementary therapies and befriending services to patients and family in the area. These organizations rely on donations to continue their efforts.

Cancer research is also a vital aspect that we can all support directly. As a matter of fact, by buying this book you have already helped – 10 percent of book royalties will be donated to support cancer research. Today, the media tells us that one third of the population may develop cancer. Research, self-healing and awareness can make those sound bytes irrelevant.

If you would like to make a donation to cancer research or to patient outreach programs, please visit the links below. Thank you for your help!

- Tufts University School of Medicine
  https://tuftsgiving.org

- Cancer Research UK
  http://www.cancerresearchuk.org/

- Community Cancer Center
  http://www.communitycancercentre.com

- McMillan Cancer Support
  http://www.macmillan.org.uk/Donate/

Appendix 1
Guided Meditations

Purifying and Relaxing Meditation
Intent: Promote relaxation and harmony in the physical body

Sit down in a quiet and comfortable place. Bring your attention to your breathing and observe its natural pace. As you breathe in, you take in healing energy from the universe. On the out breath, let go of all of the tension in your life. Sit quietly, close your eyes and listen to your breathing.

Take a deep breath in, hold it, and release. Another deep breath in, and release. Let your breath go back to its normal pace and breathe in purifying white light. Breathe out excess energy and waste. As you breathe in, your lungs fill up with life force. As you breathe out, your body lets go of every last toxin. Take another deep breath in, and relax …

Next we will scan the body and let go of any tension from the week.

Start by focusing on your feet and your ankles. Are they holding tension? Release and relax. Take your attention to your calves, release any tension and let it fall through the floor.

Moving up your thighs, lower back and hips, continue to release and relax.

Now focus on your abdomen, the digestive system and your other organs. Fill them with purifying white light, and relax. Feel your shoulders, neck and arms. Give them permission to release all tension and stress.

Take another deep breath, hold it and release. Visualize and feel an energy massage going from the top of your head to the soles of your feet.

Bring your attention back to your breathing. Breathe in, then breathe out slowly. Focus on your grounding and bring yourself back to the room.

Universal Color Meditation

Intent: Heal and release emotions and energy from the body

Note: This meditation can be used on the Aura, any of the Chakras and the physical body. It can also be used on the tumor to identify, heal and release any stuck emotions or hurts.

Sit down in a quiet and comfortable place. Bring your attention to your breathing and observe its natural pace. As you breathe in, you take in healing energy from the universe. On the out breath, let go of all of the tension in your life.

Bring your attention to your Heart Chakra as it fills up with green healing light. This light fills you with comfort, warmth and love. Stay with this throughout the meditation and let your intuition guide you through the rest.

Now bring your attention to your body/Aura/Chakra. How does it feel? Is there a particular area that you would like to heal today? Let your intuition guide you.

Ask your body to show you a color. Go with the first color that comes to mind. Is it a solid color? What does it feel like? Is it light, heavy, breezy? Slow?

Now ask the color to tell you how it feels. There are no right or wrong answers, everything is valid and deserves to be heard with love and compassion.

Thank the color for opening up to you. See and feel it filling with white or pink light. This light gently dissolves the color and releases it from your body. Bless it with love and forgiveness. Stay with this as long as you like.

Next we will fill the space with liquid gold. This gold light has the highest vibration of any energy. Visualize it filling any holes and sealing your energy.

Once the space is warm and full of gold, let that gold light trickle down through your Crown Chakra and gently fill your body, your Chakras and your Aura.

Sit with this for a few minutes and bask in the warm gold light.

Bring your attention back to your breath as it settles into its natural rhythm. Feel the weight of the chair beneath you; the soles of your feet. Take your time and slowly bring your attention to the room.

When you are ready open your eyes.

Angelic Stress Relief Meditation
Intent: Relieve stress by clearing the Solar Plexus and Heart Chakras

Sit down in a quiet and comfortable place. Bring your attention to your breathing, observing its natural pace.

Take a deep breath in, hold ... and release. Repeat this process three times, holding your breath only as long as it feels comfortable.

Let your breathing go back to its normal rhythm.

Bring your attention to your Heart Chakra: the center of unconditional love. The Heart is also the seat of your intuition and natural healing ability. Breathe gold healing light into your heart and release. Repeat this process at your own pace.

See and feel that loving energy overflow from your heart.

Now place your hands on your Solar Plexus, just below the sternum. On the next breath visualize green and gold light reaching your Solar Plexus. Visualize and feel the light clearing and balancing the energy in your Solar Plexus. The healing light fades and we are left with a bright yellow Chakra spinning beautifully.

Hold that image in your mind and feel the Chakra growing stronger.

Next we are going to release our worries by placing them in an Angel Box. By placing our fears in this box we hand them over to the Angels.

Visualize a beautiful gold box in front of you. What does it look like? Does it have intricate designs on the side? Imagine how it feels to hold it. Let it come to life.

Visualize the box opening as you place all of your fearful thoughts, worries and concerns in its gold center. Put everything that has been weighing on your mind in that box, even the thoughts that you do not admit to yourself.

This box is a gift from Archangel Michael, who gives us courage, and from Archangel Raphael, the healing angel. Imagine the box filling with gold and green angelic light. This light transmutes your thoughts and worries into positive energy.

When you open it, you see gold rays emanating from the box. Thank the angels for taking your worries and looking after you and your loved ones.

Sit with this feeling of gratitude for as long as you like.

When you are ready, bring your attention back to your breath. Feel the weight of the chair under you and slowly bring yourself back to the room.

Take as much time as you need. When you are ready, open your eyes.

Aura Cleansing Meditation
Intent: Clear the Aura of any thoughts, stress or tension

Sit down in a quiet and comfortable place. Bring your attention to your breathing and observe its natural pace. As you breathe in, you take in healing energy from the universe. As you breathe out, let go of any stress from your life.

Bring your attention to your Heart Chakra, the seat of unconditional love and compassion. As you breathe in, visualize your lungs filling with healing light.

Next we will work on clearing the Aura:

Visualize a bubble of light around your body. It extends an arm's length in any direction. Sense the color, shape and energy in the bubble. How does it feel?

See and feel pink and violet light filling the bubble with love. This infusion clears and mobilizes any stagnant energy in your auric field. It flows freely.

Check for any colors or sensations that seem out of place. Send pink and violet light to purify the energy. The light transmutes and releases the energy.

Next, visualize a long grounding cord dropping from your Base Chakra, at the root of your spine, into the earth. This cord lets energy flow down to the center of the earth where it is cleansed and purified.

Watch from a place of security as gravity sends your worries, cares and concerns to the center of the earth for purification. Release the cord and let it slip to the center of the earth as well.

Next we will fill the space left in your Aura with gold. This liquid gold light has the highest vibration of any healing energy. It fills your Aura with the healing power of love and seals it in a protective bubble of gold light.

When your Aura is completely covered, let that gold light trickle down through your Crown Chakra and gently fill your body and your Chakras.

Stay with this image as long as you need to. Rest assured in the knowledge that this gold light will continue to protect and heal you.

When you are ready, bring your attention back to your breath. Feel the weight of the chair under you and slowly bring yourself back to the room.

Take as much time as you need. When you are ready, open your eyes.

Chakra Meditation
Intent: Clear, balance and heal the Chakras

Sit down in a quiet and comfortable place. Bring your attention to your breathing and observe its natural pace. As you breathe in, you take in healing energy from the universe. As you breathe out, let go of any stress.

Place your hand over the Chakra that you wish to heal. If it is not comfortable to do so then bring your attention to that part of your body.

Get a sense of how it feels. Do you notice any colors, sensations or intuitive feelings? What do they mean? Let your intuition answer the question.

Visualize the Chakra filling with white or pink light. This light smoothes the edges and dissolves any shadows, patches or colors that you may have noticed.

Next we will fill that Chakra with liquid gold. This liquid gold is unconditional love. It heals the Chakra and raises its vibration to the highest level possible, filling every last inch of space.

Now see and feel the gold rays of light emanating from the Chakra and filling your body, especially the nearby organs and tissues. This gold light purifies, heals and balances the energy in your body. It carries the energy of love.

Sit with this for a few minutes.

Bring your attention back to the Chakra. This gold healing light starts to fade and instead we find the Chakra full of its natural color.

Use your inner voice to speak to your Chakra, telling it that you will continue to love and care for it. This sends a message to your subconscious, a signal of your commitment to play an active part in your healing process.

When you are ready, bring your attention back to your breath. Feel the weight of the chair under you and bring your attention back to the room.

Take as much time as you need. When you are ready, open your eyes.

Violet Flame Meditation

Intent: Shrink the tumor, and dissolve the emotion that it holds.

Note! If it is difficult for the Healee to visualize the tumor, the Healer can run through this mentally during the healing without verbalizing the words.

Sit down in a comfortable chair, relax and close your eyes. Feel the ground under your feet and the weight of the chair. Take a deep breath in, hold it, and release it. Visualize pink healing color in the air; as you breathe in, the pink fills your lungs. And exhale.

Repeat this breathing exercise two times.

On the inhale this energy fills your lungs, where it is infused into your bloodstream. The pink healing energy is pumped from your heart to the rest of your body. It travels through your veins and your capillaries to every last cell in your body, healing and regenerating as it goes.

Stay with this image for 2-5 minutes.

Next we are going to use visualization to release and heal the energy of the cancer cells. I would like you to bring your attention to the tumor. Start by visualizing a healing light around the tumor; it surrounds and isolates the tumor's energy from the rest of the body. The healing light is filled with energy of love and forgiveness, and it engulfs every last cell in the tumor.

Note: Sit with this image for a few minutes or as long as needed.

It is now time to purify and release the energy in the tumor. We will start by imagining a solid pink light around the tumor, containing its energy. Now visualize a violet flame in the center of the tumor. It burns with a steady healing light and consumes every last bit of the tumor's energy.

Devoid of air and energy, the cancer cells lose force. The pink light contains its energy as the tumor becomes smaller. Keep your heart centered in love and your mind focused on that violate flame until it fades away.

Note: Wait for the client to be ready.

Bring your attention back to the soles of your feet and breathe in and out slowly. You are surrounded in pink healing energy and it continues to fill your lungs on the inhale. Breathe in and out at your own pace, filling your lungs, your torso and your limbs with pink energy.

Visualize yourself in a bubble of protective white light with your guardian angels behind you and a team of healing angels circling over your head. Thank them for their healing presence and know that they will be with you until your next meditation.

Bring your attention to the muscles in your feet, your legs and your bottom. Feel the weight of the chair under you and slowly bring your attention back into the room.

Have a stretch and drink water, if you need it.

Note: This meditation is not a substitute for medical care. It should only be used in addition to the treatment recommended by your doctor. The intent is to shrink the tumor by releasing the energy of resentment and anger. My theory is that this can also be used to prevent reappearance of tumors after surgery and to assist radiation and chemotherapies in their progress.

Meditation to Energize T-Cells
Intent: Channel the energy of love and forgiveness to the tumor

Biology Note: The T-cells are the body's natural defense system. This meditation is based on the intuitive hunch that our body has a learning curve when it comes to cancer. It needs to recognize that cell as abnormal, and react. This meditation helps by infusing the T-cells with the healing qualities of love and forgiveness.

Sit down, relax and close your eyes. Take a deep breath in, hold it, and release. Visualize a pink or green healing light in the air around you. As you take your next breath this color fills your lungs.

Now breathe in and visualize that pink or green light traveling down to your Heart Chakra. On the exhale, releases any worries to the universe.

Repeat this process at your own pace.

Breathe the color in and out, releasing any tension you may have from your day. This healing color fills your lungs, your heart, and your veins. The healing light flows through your veins to every last cell in your body, purifying and healing as it goes.

Visualize the white light flowing through your bones down to the very center where your immune system is housed. The soft cartilage in the center of our bones produces the T-cells, which are our body's natural anti-bodies. These cells are intelligent; they are able to travel through the blood to help the body self-heal. Visualize and feel your T-cells filling up with the healing power of love.

Now direct the T-cells to the area where the tumor sits, and watch as they approach the tumor and surround it with the energy of love and forgiveness. They gently envelop the tumor, filling it with love, forgiveness and compassion.

The loving energy in your T-cells dissolves the tumor. It slowly starts to fade away, along with any fear, doubt or anger that you may have felt. Only love remains.

Bring your attention back to the organ where the tumor sat. Fill it with pink healing light, full of love and compassion, and release. That healing light will continue to release loving energy long after this meditation is over.

Bring your attention back to the soles of your feet, your knees and your hips. Visualize yourself breathing in light. Breathe out any traces of tension.

Visualize yourself in a bubble of protective white light with your guardian angels behind you, and a team of healing angels circling over your head. Welcome their healing presence and know that their healing energy will stay with you until your next meditation.

Slowly bring yourself back in to the room, stretch and drink water, if you need to.

Appendix 2
Glossary

The Aura is the energy field surrounding the human body. All of our thoughts, emotions, feelings and reactions are stored in the Aura.

The Brow Chakra is the energy center at the forehead. The Brow is linked to our thinking capabilities, analytical skills and intuitive vision. Related organs: eyes and brain. Its color, indigo.

The Chakras are our personal energy centers. They regulate the flow of energy in the physical, emotional, mental and spiritual body. Each of the major Chakras relates to a specific area in our life: spirituality, sight, communication, love, power, relationships and security.

The Crown Chakra is the energy center situated at the crown of the head. A clear Crown enables us to receive intuitive messages and guidance. Related organs: brain, eyes, central nervous system. Its color, violet.

Channeling is the process of drawing on universal healing energy and sharing it with others. Healers channel energy through their Heart Chakras.

Energy Healing is a complementary therapy that involves clearing and healing imbalances on the physical, emotional, mental and spiritual levels.

Epigenetics is a branch of genetics that studies the relationship between environmental signals and gene selection at the cellular level.

A Healer is a person who channels healing energy. There are natural healers who are able to channel energy with minimal training, as well as qualified healers who study energy healing for months or even years.

The Healee is the person who receives Energy Healing or Reiki.

The Heart Chakra is the energy center that enables us to give and receive love. We can send healing to any organ through the Heart. Related organs: heart, cardiovascular system, lungs, immune system and breast. Its color, green or pink.

Guided Visualizations are relaxation techniques that involve mentally seeing and feeling a sequence of events. For example: "Visualize yourself walking by the beach. Listen to the waves. Feel the sand under you toes."

Meditation involves focusing the mind on a thought, idea or concept. This can include observing the breath, repeating a mantra or bringing your attention to a particular concept, object (e.g., a candle) or a mental picture.

Memes are learned behaviors and beliefs that spread through observation and imitation. They are often part of shared identities in families and tribes.

Reiki is a Japanese healing technique that relies on universal spiritual energy to restore mental, emotional, spiritual and physical imbalances. Practitioners need to be attuned to Reiki by a Reiki Master.

The Root Chakra is located at the base of the spine. It relates to our feelings of vitality, safety and community. It is also linked to the physical Aura layer. Related organs: skeleton, skin and bowels. Its color, red.

The Sacral Chakra is the energy center below the navel. It is linked to our creative drive, passion and our relationships. Related organs: bladder, kidneys and female reproductive organs. Its color, orange.

The Solar Plexus Chakra is the energy center in upper stomach. It is the seat of our personal power and reflects self-esteem. Related organs: stomach, liver, spleen, and digestive system. Its color, yellow.

The Throat Chakra is the energy center at the throat. The Throat governs our ability to communicate our thoughts, feelings and emotions. Related organs: throat, ears, thyroid, esophagus and neck. Its color, light blue.

Appendix 3
Energy Management for Beginners

The following has been taken from the Energy Basics page on my blog. This information will be helpful for novice Healers who are opening up to channel energy. It includes simple techniques that can be used to ground, protect and cleanse your energy on a daily basis. These steps are helpful for those of us who want to give healing regularly.

What is Healing?

The dictionary defines healing as:

1. to make healthy, whole, or sound: restore to health: free from ailment.
2. to bring to an end or conclusion, as conflicts between people or groups, usually with the strong implication of restoring former amity; settle; reconcile: *They tried to heal the rift between them but were unsuccessful.*
3. to ... cleanse, purify: *to heal the soul*

How does this apply to me?

Raise your hand if you have ever thought stress was responsible for your aches and pains. If so, you might like to try one of the following relaxation techniques:

Journaling, talking, **laughing**, meditating, sharing, spending time with friends, **hugging**, smiling, being smiled at, cuddling, **singing**, dancing, **laughing**, laughing, more laughing, **breathing exercises**, walking, **skiing**, cycling, sailing, fishing, yoga, **meditation**, etc.

What is Energy Healing?

Energy Healing is a complementary therapy that includes healing of the physical, emotional, mental and spiritual aspects. Healers work by channeling universal energy through their body to the Healee. This can help release mental, emotional and spiritual blocks or imbalances that may be holding them back. It is complementary to medical care, not alternative.

Grounding Your Energy

An adrenalin rush is an overflow of energy. Though these bursts of energy are not so common in our daily lives, we do sometimes feel them after a healing session. As a novice or student Healer, there may be times when you will feel yourself buzzing or even a bit frazzled. We can regulate our personal energy levels by sending excess energy into the ground through the Chakras on the soles of your feet. A regular grounding practice can also strengthen the energy body.

The following is a simple grounding meditation:

Visualize yourself at the foot of an oak tree. See and feel the earth under your feet and the trunk at your back. The weight of the tree keeps you in a comfortable and stable position. The weather is calm and reassuring. Breathe in and out slowly, observing the natural rhythm of your body.

Bring your attention to the soles of your feet. Visualize roots growing out of the bottom of your feet and sinking into the earth. They are as strong as the tree's roots. They draw on the natural moisture, nutrients and water in the earth. Drawing on these roots will strengthen your energy. *

Note: This meditation is only for the Healer. In healing school we were taught that earth energy is not helpful for cancer patients because it has a tendency to make things grow. When we channel energy to the cancer patient we only use universal spiritual energy, such as Reiki or white light.

For more on grounding please visit www.healingforgrounding.com

Clearing Your Energy

Clearing our energy enables us to let go of any feelings or emotions that we may have absorbed from others. This can be done by visualizing a shower of white light running through your Aura. It is best practice to clear our energy field daily and certainly after each healing session. This clears and releases any feelings that we may have absorbed from other people. An energetic cleanse is a quick way to feel refreshed and energized. This can also be done to clear your mind.

Center in The Heart

Most of us tend to center our energy in a particular Chakra. This is linked to our behavior. Those of us with a tendency to think things through and analyze everything are usually centered in the Brow Chakra. Those who hold their energy in the Solar Plexus might be very outgoing. Those who speak out often and voice their opinions may be centered in the Throat.

Many schools of thought point to the Heart as the ideal place to be centered. The Heart Chakra is the midway point between the Crown, which gives us access to our intuition and the Root Chakra, which keeps us grounded in reality. When we are centered in the Heart we can also access the Throat and Brow Chakras from a place of love, compassion and security. This makes it easier to see life clearly and to voice our opinions in an open, honest and loving manner.

Energetic Protection

Though working on ourselves from a spiritual and energetic point of view can be very empowering, it can also make us more susceptible to other people's vibes. We come into contact with other people's energy at work, in public and also in one-to-one interactions. It is usually harmless, though if you are a naturally sensitive person you may start to feel these energies intensely. There were a few months when I saw a crowd and wanted to run the other way. Since then I have discovered psychic or energetic protection and this is no longer a problem.

Here are a few tips. Most of them involve visualization and intention.

- Take a moment to visualize a bubble of white, pink or violet light enveloping your aura. The light goes over your head, under your feet and about 1.5 feet on your front and back. The boundaries are strong enough to contain your energy. Anything that hits the edge of the bubble slides or bounces off. I also like to imagine a vacuum cleaner that catches anything negative around me and sends it back to the universe to be purified.

- This is a personal favorite: visualize a long wizard cloak, like the ones from Harry Potter. It can be any color you like as long as it reaches the floor and covers your head. The material is very flexible so it is easy to walk in, but it is strong and heavy enough to offer real protection. You can also make it an invisible cloak if you like.

- Asking for protection is also fantastic, especially if you believe in angels. The name that comes to mind is Archangel Michael. He is a warrior angel, and looks after light workers, servicemen and armies.

- Now onto intention and trust. Regardless of the method chosen, intend for it to work and trust you are safe, protected and free.

Grounding, Centering and Protecting

Now that we have mastered the individual steps, it is time to do them in one go. With a little practice the whole process takes no longer than five minutes. It is worth doing this daily as part of an energy hygiene routine. It might even help to run through this after your daily shower.

- Ground yourself by bringing your attention to your feet.
- Visualize a shower of white light clearing your auric field.
- Bring your attention to your heart chakra.
- Visualize a protective bubble of light – and off you go!

Appendix 4

Recommended Reading

Books have been a big part of my life from early childhood. For years I read nothing but fiction, devouring everything from Anne of Green Gables, to Dickens and Harry Potter. Then I moved onto self-help books, especially on Energy Healing, Kabbalah and intuition. These have shaped the way I approach relationships and life in general. After a few months I had enough of reading and found a school that taught them in more detail.

The past three years I have studied at the London College of Psychic Studies. Initially, I was curious and a bit skeptical. We can all develop our intuition. The difficult part is trusting the images and interpreting them accurately. In parallel, I enrolled in a two-year course in Energy Healing at the School of Intuition and Healing. As I am writing this book, my formal healing studies have come to an end. This book covers the aspects relevant to cancer. The following list should help if you wish to take healing further:

Schools for Healing and Intuition

- http://www.DiaryofaPsychicHealer.com (Online)
- http://www.intuitionandhealing.co.uk/ (UK)
- http://www.collegeofpsychicstudies.co.uk/ (UK)
- http://www.harryedwards.org.uk/ (UK)
- http://www.barbarabrennan.com/ (US & Austria)
- http://www.universityofsantamonica.edu/ (US)
- www.reiki-meditation.co.uk (UK)

Books on Self-Healing

- *The Essence of Self-Healing* by Petrene Soames
- *You Can Heal Your Life* by Louise Hay
- *Anatomy of the Spirit* by Caroline Myss
- *The Power of Healing Prayer* by Richard McAlear
- *Love, Medicine and Miracles* by Bernie Siegel

Books for student healers

- *Hands of Light* by Barbara Brennan
- *Reiki for Life* by Penelope Quest
- *The Aura and the Chakras an Owner's Manual* by Karla McLaren

Books on Angels and Psychic Development

- *Chakra Healing & Magick* by Regina Chouza
- *Psychic Development Simplified* by Wojciech "Nathaniel" Usarzewicz
- *Angel Therapy Cards* by Doreen Virtue

About The Author

Regina Chouza is a Reiki Master and Energy Healer with a BA in Philosophy from Tufts University. In 2012 she left a successful career in the corporate world to become a Healer. Regina was a continuing student at the College of Psychic Studies (2009-2013) and the School of Intuition and Healing where she studied the Mind-Body-Spirit connection.
Visit her blog at www.diaryofapsychichealer.com

65372367R00060

Made in the USA
Middletown, DE
26 February 2018